ACCENT MODIFICATION MANUAL

MATERIALS AND ACTIVITIES

ACCENT MODIFICATION MANUAL

MATERIALS AND ACTIVITIES

Harold T. Edwards, Ph.D.
Kathy Harris Strattman, M.A.
Wichita State University
Wichita, Kansas

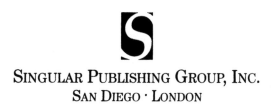

SINGULAR PUBLISHING GROUP, INC.
SAN DIEGO · LONDON

Singular Publishing Group, Inc.
4284 41st Street
San Diego, California 92105-1197

19 Compton Terrace
London, N1 2UN, United Kingdom
5 6 7 8 9 10 NET/NET 9 8 7 6 5
© 1996 Singular Publishing Group, Inc.

Typeset in 11/13 ITC Century Schoolbook by So Cal Graphics
Printed in the United States of America by McNaughton & Gunn

ISBN 1-56593-453-9

CONTENTS

FOREWORD

Juan sapon atain huas tri lirel pigues. De espen ola deirtain bilding dijaus for tulivin. Neber deytak di siestas. Ola tain huorc, huorc, huorc. Estupid pigues! Ar mucha bera zing turu liac eslip. If hiugarra du somzin, iz bera tudo dat. Bot dis pigues quipon huorquin . . .

Author Unknown

Literal Translation:

Once upon a time was three little pigs. They spend all of their time building the house for to live in. Never they take the siestas. All of their time work, work, work. Stupid pigs! A much better thing to do like sleep. If we gotta do something, is better to do that. But these pigs keep on working . . .

We all sound strange to somebody. People today talk a lot about the accents, dialects, and world Englishes they hear. Language differences pique everyone's curiosity and alert us to our larger world. We may have already begun to notice that English no longer belongs to those of us who grew up speaking it, but rather to millions of others, struggling daily with its awkward spelling and pronunciation.

These days no one doubts that English has, at least for the next millennium, taken its place on the world stage as the medium for global communication. When a Haitian greets a Guatemalan, an Arab buys a car from an Australian or sells oil to a Ugandan, a Japanese student registers in an American university, or a Vietnamese refugee negotiates getting the electricity turned on, Englishes are spoken. When, however, these individuals' accents (Englishes) deviate too far from standard versions, the message may be lost. The curtain comes down mid-script as the actors fail to execute the scene.

A By-Product No More

Many in the field perceive pronunciation as a by-product of the language learning process, rather than an overt objective. The innovative curricular approach of this text, however, brings accent modification forward as a type of language study in its own right. I believe this text is at the cusp of a changing view about pronunciation teaching, though ESL/EFL teachers are not always eager to change their ways. This manual creatively breaks new ground and, without a doubt, fills a glaring gap in this slowly evolving field.

The Predicament

Nonnative speakers frequently face great frustration in everyday interactions when they are not understood. Learners are nipping at the heels of teachers, demanding strategies that will allow them to get through their daily communication ordeals. Such language learners are almost universally aware of their predicament, but totally at a loss about how to fix it. Usually their teachers are, too. Attempts to learn more grammar or more words only compound the problem because language is much more than rules and words. Birdwhitsell (1970) and Mehrabian and Ferris (1967) suggest that words represent less than 30% of communication. The rest is voice, tone, and kinesics. The case for this book is thus made. Its focus is prosody which is central to pronunciation. This text, more astutely than any I have seen, advances this notion and offers students a road map for maneuvering around and through that complex phenomenon.

A Perplexing Mystery

Have you ever asked yourself how people end up with such jarring and often unintelligible accents? In some respects, this is not a mystery. Consider that

- ■ Teachers may speak English with a heavy accent;

- ■ Learners may have been taught the language through grammar-translation or reading, and have had little or no opportunity to hear or speak the language;

- ■ Learners' first languages may be phonologically at opposite ends of the spectrum from English;

- ■ The demand on learners to use English may outstrip their abilities—often a result of early and constant immersion into the target culture with insufficient language preparation (Higgs & Clifford, 1982);

- ■ Learners may not erroneously believe that language learning is about memorizing words and sentences apart from pronunciation; and

- ■ Learners may not have a "good ear" for the sounds and melodies of the target language.

Why some learners end up with convoluted accents is still quite a mystery. Aside from the nebulous notion of first language transfer (i.e., the patterns of a learner's first language carry over and influence the patterns of the second language), neither linguists nor neurolinguists can tell us enough about the process of second language acquisition to explain satisfactorily why some individuals are intelligible and others are not.

From Pattern to Meaning

This text helps students use their cognitive and problem-solving abilities to examine the key elements of the intonation system of American English, how it is organized and, more importantly, how it works in communication. Students are given the tools, the kinesthetic practice of "diagramming" pitch changes, to learn to recognize patterns of intonation (e.g., walk, jump, step, fall). After all, isn't recognizing patterns and then creating meaning out of those patterns essential to learning a language?

Pronunciation in Context

Context is to pronunciation as location is to the establishment of a new business. Learners have to understand how pronunciation and context come together to create authentic communication. Language context will come alive as learners use this text and participate in the communication activities (e.g., *What should you say?* in Lesson 6, the *Focused Interview* in Lesson 7, *Show and Tell* in Lesson 8, and *Who am I?* in Lesson 11). These kinds of bridging activities are pivotal in creating the all-important context for learning another language. This book offers learners a series of ever greater challenges in its compendium of well-developed, field-tested, solo and interactive exercises that guide students with deft precision toward the goal of modifying their accents, becoming more intelligible, or simply gaining personal confidence through a knowledge of accent modification strategies.

The Long Haul

The strategies in this text provide the framework for the long haul, for the life-long process of modifying an accent. Since learners profiles differ, they may have to focus on different aspects of the modification process. The *Accent Modification Agreement* (Appendix B) is an especially creative way of engaging learners in the process, and eliciting ownership of and a commitment to their own personalized improvement plan.

Though the exercises allow for individual differences and emphases, I like the notion that the book nonetheless has a crystal clear focus and does not try to accomplish everything about speaking American English. This well-defined focus has the effect of offering hope to learners that they can, in fact, modify their own accents as they become more and more comfortable with the doable techniques presented. The authors have succeeded in bringing together the traditional knowledge base regarding American English pronunciation and a refreshingly ample set of new strategies for learners to use.

All in all, this book strikes an impressive balance between didactics and activities, process and product, theory and practice. By reading and studying this volume it may render null and void your excuses for not learning—or teaching—more intelligible pronunciation.

Peggy J. Anderson, Ph.D.
Director TESOL Programs
Wichita State University

References

Birdwhitsell, R. (1970). *Kinesics and context*. Philadelphia: University of Pennsylvania Press.

Higgs, T., & Clifford, R. (1982). The push toward communication. In T. Higgs (Ed.), *Curriculum, competence, and the foreign language teacher* (pp. 57–79). Stokie, IL: National Textbook Company.

Mehrabian, A., & Ferris, S. (1967). Inference of attitudes from nonverbal communication in two channels. *Journal of Consulting Psychology, 31*(3), 248–252.

PREFACE

No text with its roots in pedagogy stands alone as the sole contribution of its authors. This is especially true of a text on the pronunciation of American English. Influences found in these pages stretch from the germinal work of Charles Fries, Robert Lado, John Catford, and Mary Finocchiaro, to the more recent endeavor of Larry Selinker, Joan Morley, Mary Temperley, and Rita Wong, for example.

Yet no one has had greater motivational impact on this text than David Stern whose influence began at the time he was a colleague at Wichita State University. His theoretical foundations in prosody have contributed greatly to our pedagogical and research efforts—and ultimately to the motivation for writing this text. Obviously, the departures that we have made from his conceptual framework are ours alone. Nevertheless, David Stern deserves credit for changing our approach from total emphasis on sound production to the broader and more important emphasis on prosody.

In addition, a pronunciation text requires contributions from many knowledgeable associates on the local scene. Peggy Anderson, Mary Gordon-Brannan, Tom Kneil, Rae Cuda, Suzanne Graham, Pete Krause, and Michael Pilcher provided valuable assistance in conducting the supporting research on which the concepts set forth in this text is based.

We also thank the following graduate students who have participated in field testing and evaluating these materials: Debbe Jantz, Paige Keithly, Connie Loran, Lin McGregor, Barbara Pagel, Marguerite Pangelinan, Wendy Prater, Haley Pringle, Jerry Smartt, Mary Caitlin Smith, Darlene Stokes, Janette Warne, Homer Welker, and Beth White. Julie Scherz assisted in adapting the text to individual use in the clinical setting. We are grateful for the critical assessment and encouragement that we have received from these student-colleagues.

We wish to thank Mark Allen and Judy Dillard for their highly competent and professional technical assistance. The graphics were made possible by the creative work of Jeremy Gadbury, Dale Strattman, Tom Kneil, Brian Hand, and Andy Strattman.

A special note of appreciation is also in order to the exceptional staff at Singular Publishing Group—especially, Marie Linvill, Sandy Doyle, and Angie Singh—for their high quality editorial support.

Finally, we would like to thank our many students from around the world who have participated in and contributed to the development of these materials. Their success in speaking American English has served to motivate our efforts and it is to them that we dedicate this text.

LESSON 1

Getting Ready to Speak American English

OBJECTIVE

Before we begin any serious activity, we must first develop a positive philosophy that will direct our action. In this lesson, we will state some general principles essential to a personal philosophy about *accent modification*.

GENERAL PRINCIPLES

Accent modification refers to any change that a person makes in *speaking* another language. It is different from *learning* English as another language. In the general study of English, we learn to read, write, and comprehend without much attention to speaking. In accent modification, we emphasize speaking without much emphasis on the other components of the language. You probably already have a working knowledge of the grammar of American English and are able to read and understand the language well. Your goal in studying accent modification is to acquire control of speaking so that others will understand you better. For many individuals, speaking to be understood is their major goal. It is not unusual for people to live in another country for years without gaining control of this important component of the language.

Before beginning to modify an accent, we must develop a philosophy—a positive and realistic way of thinking about accent modification. As you work on your personal philosophy, there are several important things to keep in mind. Here is a list of practical suggestions.

■ Changing speech is interesting but difficult; it takes time and effort.

Learning to speak understandably does not happen overnight. There is no magic potion, no pill, and no easy method. Only with time and effort can we make the progress we desire. Fortunately, many students find this process fun and interesting. They actually enjoy the hard work because they are able to see the value of the changes they are making. People understand them better, and that is sufficient reward for all the hours spent practicing.

In learning to speak another language, certain features of pronunciation are important. When these features are the same as those in our native language, there may be little problem. However, when these forms of pronunciation are very different or when they conflict with what we know, they can become serious obstacles that take time and effort to modify.

■ Although the sounds of language are important, success in accent modification is not obtained by knowledge about sounds.

Students frequently believe that good speech results from "learning about" speech sounds. Although this information is interesting, it will not result in much change in your accent. There is not enough time during the actual process of speaking to remember how to produce all the sounds in the new language. By the time we have thought about what we are going to say and have selected the words and the proper grammar to use, there is no time to think about sounds. Unfortunately, no one has ever learned to speak another language fluently by studying its sounds.

■ It is not necessary to speak exactly like a native speaker of American English to be understood or to have good speech.

A student once said, "I'm not going to speak English until I can speak it perfectly." Obviously, this student missed the point of accent modification and also missed wonderful opportunities to communicate with many people because of an impractical goal. What is "perfect" English? There is no general agreement. No two speakers of a language speak exactly the same. We cannot say that one is more perfect than the other. Our goal is to be understood, not to have perfect speech. The student should have said, "I'm going to practice speaking English until I can be understood perfectly."

■ **Learn to listen and watch. Native speakers can teach us about American English by the *way they speak* and *what they do* when they speak.**

Learn to be a listener and an observer of people when they talk. Try to select opportunities in which you do not have to listen to what people are saying, but can concentrate on the way they are speaking. Turn off the sound on a television set and watch the movements as people talk. Then, with the sound on, turn away from the picture and listen to the way they talk. Become a student of facial movement and vocal expression.

■ **Experiment! If the way you usually speak sounds understandable to you, it may not be understandable to others; if it sounds natural to you, it may sound unnatural to others.**

All progress is the result of experimentation. We need to consider our work in accent modification as a laboratory for trying some different things. You will learn to make some modifications that will make your speech more understandable. Don't be afraid of changes that make speech understandable. Be afraid of continuing as before without modifying your accent. When you speak so that others understand, they appreciate your effort to help them.

WHAT CHANGING YOUR SPEECH WILL *NOT* CHANGE

■ **Accent modification will not change identity or personality.**

Every speaker has a particular way of speaking so that no two speakers of a language will sound exactly the same. This individualized manner of speaking is the result of all kinds of influences from family, friends, teachers, and even from the way our vocal tracts are made. Even when people change their accent, their *voices* will not change. Students sometimes think they will not sound like themselves if they modify their accent.

As we will see in Lesson 2, there are certain things that we can modify in our speech, but we will never lose our identity. Once again, the purpose of accent modification is to make your speech more understandable, nothing else. The changes that we make in accent modification do not affect our voices, only the way we use our voices to speak.

Changing the way you speak American English will not change your personality either. There is nothing in this method that will alter who you are. If you are friendly, creative, or fun to be with, for example, you will continue to be as you are. In fact, when your English-speaking friends begin to understand you better and stop asking you to repeat, the "real you" might even be seen more clearly.

REMEMBER YOUR LISTENER

■ **The "golden rule" of accent modification is to speak to your listener the way you want your listener to speak to you.**

We modify our accent, not for ourselves, but so that others can understand us better. Although some changes may be difficult and require considerable effort, there are several things that we can remember to do from the very beginning.

1. Wait until you have finished talking to laugh or smile.

We all want to be friendly, and some things that we say are humorous. Yet you should wait until you have finished speaking before you laugh, or wait until you have finished laughing before you speak. Laughter and smiling cause a distortion of the mouth. It is almost impossible to speak clearly when you are smiling or laughing.

2. Let your listener see your face.

Try not to cover your face or turn your head while you are talking. It is very helpful for your listener to see your face when you speak because it helps your listener "to see" what you are saying.

3. Speak to be heard.

We all need to speak loudly enough to be understood. The situation will determine what loudness level we should use. When speaking to a group, we will use a louder voice than when we are talking to one or two other persons.

REVIEW OF GENERAL PRINCIPLES FOR ACCENT MODIFICATION

1. Changing speech is interesting but difficult; it takes time and effort.

2. Although the sounds of language are important, success in accent modification is not obtained by knowledge about sounds.

3. It is not necessary to speak exactly like a native speaker of American English to be understood or to have good speech.

4. Learn to listen and watch. Native speakers can teach us about American English by the *way they speak* and *what they do* when they speak. In fact, they can teach us more by what they do than by what they *tell* us they do!

5. Experiment! If the way you usually speak sounds understandable to you, it may not be understandable to others; if it sounds natural to you, it may sound unnatural to others.

6. Accent modification will not change identity or personality.

7. The "golden rule" of accent modification is to speak to your listener the way you want your listener to speak to you.

EXERCISE 1. A Personal Philosophy for Accent Modification.

Based on the material presented in this lesson, write a personal philosophy that will support your activities in accent modification. Which of these general principles will you have to remember?

_____

_____

_____

_____

_____

_____

_____

_____

_____

LESSON 2

Understanding Accent Modification

OBJECTIVE

In this lesson, you will learn:

- What American English is;

- What a *dialect* is;

- What an *accent* is;

- What *accent modification* is;

- What general adjustments are necessary for speaking American English;

- What *speech elements* are changed when we modify our accent; and

- What a *syllable* is and how it is important to speech.

WHAT IS AMERICAN ENGLISH?

Many varieties of English are spoken in the world today. In fact, English serves as a *lingua franca* or business language in many parts of the world. In England, British English is spoken, whereas in the United States, American English is used. The varieties of English may differ in vocabulary, pronunciation, and some grammatical forms, but each is recognizable as English. In this text, the standard features of spoken American English are explained and practiced.

WHAT IS A DIALECT?

In every country where a variety of English is spoken, there also may be various dialects. Just as there are dialects of British English, there are different dialects of American English in the United States. Speakers from Alabama, New York, and Oregon may sound very different from each other. We can say that they speak three different dialects of American English—*Southern American*, *Eastern American*, and *Pacific Northwest American* (Edwards, 1992).

Every speaker of a language speaks a dialect of that language. Dialects are caused by *isolation*. Geographic, political, economic, social, or cultural barriers may keep one group of people from communicating with another group of speakers of the same language. When groups of people are isolated from other groups of people, their speech will change and dialects result. Dialects only become a problem when they block easy communication between people.

WHAT IS AN ACCENT?

At times, the words dialect and accent may mean the same thing. People whose speech is different from that of the community in which they live are often said to speak with a dialect or accent, whether or not their speech represents one of the standard dialects of their language. In this text, *dialect* will be used for a standard variety of a language (Southern American, Eastern American, and Pacific Northwest American) that results from some kind of isolation.

The best word for referring to the speech of nonnative speakers of a language is *accent*. Therefore, the terms *foreign accent* and *accent modification* are preferred over *foreign dialect* and *foreign dialect modification*. A person's dialect is the result of isolation, as we have said, but a person's accent results from *transfer* or *influence* of characteristics from the native language. The way we learned to speak our native language may "transfer" to the way we speak another language.

WHAT IS ACCENT MODIFICATION?

Accent modification is a process of formal training to make the speech of a nonnative speaker of a language more understandable. The goal is not usually the

UNDERSTANDING ACCENT MODIFICATION   **9**

total elimination of a person's accent, but (1) the *reduction* of those characteristics that make the speech of the nonnative speaker difficult to understand, and (2) the *addition* of those characteristics that make speech easy to understand. In this sense, both accent reduction *and* accent addition must occur for the overall modification of speaking.

WHY IS MODIFYING AN ACCENT IMPORTANT?

The most important reason for modifying our speech is to become more understandable. Our lives are more satisfying, successful, and personally rewarding if we can speak so that others understand us. You probably have your own reasons for wanting to improve your ability to communicate in American English. Perhaps you want to get a job for which English is important or become a teacher of English as another language. The reasons for modifying an accent are as varied as the people who want to accomplish this important goal.

WHAT IS "INTERLANGUAGE ACCENT"?

Learning to speak another language is complicated by the many factors that guide the process. Some of us are better at language learning than others, some have had more experience or better instruction than others, and some are more highly motivated than others. As a result, no two learners of another language will be identical to each other or to any native speaker of that language. This variability is called *interlanguage accent* (Selinker, 1972). For example, if ten students are studying American English, there will be a different interlanguage accent of English spoken by each student in the class, and the speech of each student will be different from the form of English spoken by the teacher.

THE INTERLANGUAGE ACCENT SCALE

We can create a scale showing the variability that exists in speech. At one end is the speech that no one understands; at the other end is the speech that is completely understood all of the time.

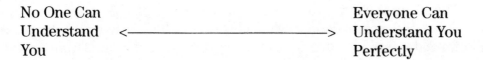

No One Can Understand You <————————————————> Everyone Can Understand You Perfectly

Where do you think *you* are on this scale? The purpose of accent modification is to assist you in improving your speech so that you can become more understandable in speaking another language, in this case, American English. Every student of American English may be on a different point on the Interlanguage Accent Scalé because it represents a broad range of speech. Where you are on this scale *now* is not very important. One person may start accent modification on the left side of the scale whereas another might begin toward the middle. Both students can set goals for improvement that will result in a move toward the right side of the scale.

PREPARING TO SPEAK AMERICAN ENGLISH: GENERAL ADJUSTMENTS

When runners prepare for a race, they select appropriate clothing, including proper shoes, and warm up by stretching their muscles. Every activity requires preliminary adjustments. Even when we write a letter, we must obtain the materials we need, find a comfortable location, and position ourselves so that arm and hand can be used efficiently. When we speak, we also need to make certain important adjustments.

1. Relaxing the Muscles of the Face

Different languages make different use of the facial muscles. For American English, the muscles of the face, especially the cheeks and upper lip, tend to be relaxed, as shown in *Figure 2–1*. When required, muscle tension usually centers on the lower lip. You should learn to relax the muscles around the mouth for better sounding American English speech. A mirror is useful in learning to control the muscles of the face.

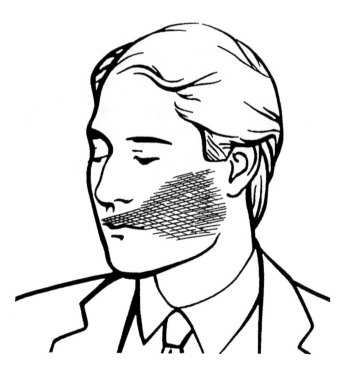

Figure 2–1. The relaxed areas of the face. The shading on the sides of the face and upper lip indicate areas that are usually relaxed during speech.

> **Pronunciation Note:** The same muscle generally makes up the upper and lower lips. When the lower lip is tensed, the upper lip may also move slightly, especially at the corners.

EXERCISE 1. Relaxing the Muscles

Look at your mouth in a mirror. Round your lips as if you were going to whistle. Then relax. Repeat this several times watching the muscles that form your lips tense and relax. The rest of your face should remain relaxed. Now, using the mirror, examine the muscles of the sides of the face and lips as you say, *Good morning. How are you today?* in your native language. Then say it again, but in English. Now answer these questions by circling *Yes* or *No* as appropriate.

Do you see any differences in the way the muscles are used?	YES	NO
Does your upper lip move when you say this in your native language?	YES	NO
Does your upper lip move when you say this in American English?	YES	NO
Does your lower lip move when you say this in your native language?	YES	NO
Does your lower lip move when you say this in American English?	YES	NO
Are the muscles of your face more relaxed when you speak your native language than when you speak American English?	YES	NO

If you found no differences, perhaps you need to work on relaxing the muscles of the face and upper lip. If you observed differences, perhaps you have already realized that American English requires a different use of muscles than many other languages.

EXERCISE 2. Observation

Observe several native speakers of American English speaking (teachers, classmates, business associates). Notice the muscle movements of the upper lip, the lower lip, and the sides of the face.

Are these muscles generally tense or relaxed?   TENSE   RELAXED

Observe several speakers of American English on television. Turn down the sound so that you can concentrate on the *way* each is speaking rather than on *what* each is saying. Observe the muscle movements of the upper lip as compared to the lower lip. Observe the sides of the face. In a few sentences, describe what you see.

_____

_____

_____

_____

_____

_____

2. Producing the Tone (Voice)

We usually speak on vibrations that come from the voice box in the throat (*Figure 2–2*). When these vibrations occur, we say that speech is *voiced*. Most speech sounds are voiced. However, some speech is spoken on air without the usual vibrations that come from the throat. This kind of speech is *voiceless*.

EXERCISE 3. Feeling the Vibrations

Say the sound /ee/ as in the word *see* while you place your fingers lightly on your throat to sense the vibration from the voice box (larynx). What you are experiencing is *voicing*. Next, pronounce the first sound of *see*—/s/. Notice that there are no vibrations from the larynx. The /s/ sound is *voiceless*.

EXERCISE 4. Selecting Voiced and Voiceless Sounds

Here are some sounds common to American English. Circle those that are made with voice box vibration and are voiced. The uncircled sounds will be voiceless because they are not produced with vibrations from the voice box. See Appendix D for a list of phonetic symbols used in this text.

Example:  /ee/   /sh/

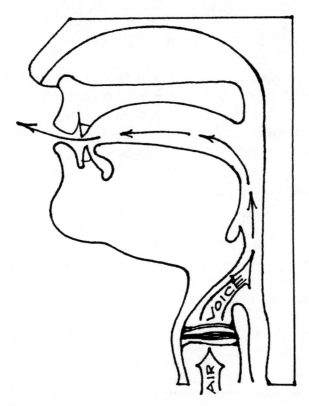

Figure 2–2. How voice is produced. Air from the lungs may create vibrations in the voice box that resonate through the remaining vocal tract to produce speech.

/s/	/m/	/p/
/o/	/f/	/b/
/v/	/h/	/u/

3. Centering the Tone (Resonance)

Every language has a preferred place in the human vocal tract around which it centers the majority of its sounds (technically known as resonance). For American English, this point is *in the center of the mouth* (Stern, 1991). In fact, the most frequent vowel sound in the language, the neutral vowel, is made in the middle of the mouth (*Figure 2–3*). Speech that is centered in front of or behind this point in the mouth may sound unnatural to native speakers of American English.

EXERCISE 5. Sensing the Tone

Place your hands, palms forward, on the sides of your face, at a point that is close to the center of the mouth. In your native language say, *Good morning. How are*

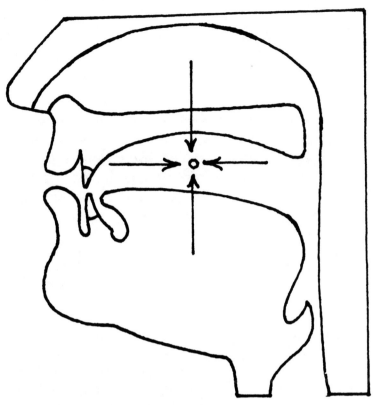

Figure 2–3. Centering the tone. Speakers of American English generally focus their speech around a point in the center of the mouth.

you today? Now repeat these phrases in English as you try to center the speech at the point marked by your hands. Can you sense a difference?

EXERCISE 6. The Neutral Vowel

The most frequent vowel in American English is called the *neutral vowel.* Your teacher will pronounce these words. Listen carefully and circle all the neutral vowels in each word.

| **Example:** | division |

| banana | maximum | delicious | umbrella |
| telegram | ballot | bishop | modification |

THE PRIMARY SPEECH ELEMENTS

Although changing the way we speak is difficult, there are some elements of speech that we can learn to control that will make speech more understandable.

Fortunately, some are more important to American English than others. These we will call the *primary speech elements*.

1. Pitch

The most important speech element in American English is pitch (Bolinger, 1986). Pitch is used for signaling the important words in speech and is considered to be the primary mechanism for *stress*. As such, it contributes to meaning in that a higher pitch is used for important words. Pitch is also related to *intonation*, the changes in melody that occur as we speak. Usually we understand better when persons sing in another language than when they speak the same words because pitch (intonation) is controlled by the music. Therefore, opera singers, who use a variety of languages, have less of an accent when they sing.

2. Rhythm

A marching band relies on the drummer to maintain the rhythm, a pattern of repeated beats, some strong and some weak that occur in time. The strong beats will be longer than the weak beats, but all the beats will occur regularly, either fast or slow as the music requires. Speech also has rhythm, a recurring pattern of fast or slow beats on long or short syllables. We call the overall timing of the syllables *rate*, and the length of the individual syllables is known as *duration*. *Pausing*, the silence between syllables, also contributes to rhythm.

- ■ **Rate.** Rate refers to how fast or slow we talk. If a person speaks too fast, people will not be able to understand. A rate that is too slow is frequently considered uninteresting. The student of American English should adopt a comfortable speaking rate for most situations.

- ■ **Duration.** Duration refers to the relative length of a syllable, usually determined by the length of the vowel. When the vowel in a syllable is lengthened, the duration of that syllable becomes longer. Some syllables in American English are longer than others. As with pitch, duration is used to stress important words. Duration is important to rhythm because it changes the timing of speech. This element will be developed more fully as you participate in the instruction provided by this text.

- ■ **Pausing.** We regularly have to pause to breathe. At other times, we may stop speaking to think of a word or to allow our listener to think about what we just said. Pauses may be planned or unplanned. In speaking American English, you will want to learn how to use planned pauses, but how to avoid unplanned pauses. Planned pauses contribute to the rhythm of our speech; unplanned pauses cause speech to be irregular and difficult to understand.

THE SECONDARY SPEECH ELEMENTS

Pitch and rhythm (rate, duration, and pausing) are the primary speech elements because they are used to signal changes in meaning more frequently than elements that serve a secondary function. As you advance in your study of American English, you will want to develop these elements to add emotional interest to what you say.

1. Loudness

Loudness refers to the intensity of speech. In a noisy room we have to speak louder than we do in a quiet room. We also have to use more loudness when we speak to groups, such as to a class, than when we speak to one other person. Some persons refer to this variable as the *volume* of speech, similar to the volume control on a radio or television set.

Speakers of some languages use loudness the way pitch is used in American English—to signal the important words. You may have to learn to reduce your dependency on loudness, especially since in American English culture loudness signals assertiveness, aggression, and anger. Teachers have to learn to increase the overall loudness of their speech without using too much loudness on individual words or syllables.

2. Quality

Certain changes can be made in the vocal tract to change the way our voices sound. For example, we may speak in a breathy voice or a nasal voice to communicate certain emotional states. The nonnative speaker of American English should use a natural voice for most communication situations. Changes in quality are difficult to learn because they are frequently related to subtle cultural factors.

VARIABLE INTERACTIONS

The speech elements—primary and secondary—may be used in combination with each other. For example, pitch can interact with loudness which may interact with rate and/or quality to produce many possibilities for communicating feelings and interpretations. Although such control is to be desired, it is better to learn the basics and leave variable interactions for a later, more advanced stage in accent modification.

THE SYLLABLE: THE BASIC UNIT OF SPEECH

It is necessary to remember that syllables are constructed out of sounds and words are constructed out of syllables. Both sounds and words are organized around the syllable. We speak in syllables, not sounds or words, and we control the syllables we speak by means of the primary and secondary speech elements. Therefore, the syllable is the basic unit of speech.

Syllables will vary in terms of

■ *Pitch*—some will be higher or lower than others;

■ *Rate*—some syllables will be faster or slower than others;

■ *Duration*—some syllables will be longer or shorter than others;

■ *Loudness*—some will be louder or softer than others; and

■ *Quality*—some syllables will be spoken with a particular vocal change to give them color or interest.

Syllables are organized into a *releasing sound,* usually called a consonant (or C) and a *melodic sound,* usually called a vowel (or V). We will learn more about the syllable and its variations in Lesson 14. For the moment, it is sufficient to view the syllable as a combination of consonant and vowel. Therefore, we speak more like this (CV means "consonant, vowel"):

CV-CV-CV, as in PO-TA-TO

than in isolated sounds like this:

SOUND-SOUND-SOUND-SOUND-SOUND-SOUND, as in

P—O—T—A—T—O

or in isolated words like this:

WORD-WORD-WORD-WORD-WORD-WORD-WORD, as in

THE-POTATO-IS-A-FOOD-EVERYONE-LIKES.

EXERCISE 7. Vowels

We have learned that syllables are made of consonants and vowels. In this exercise, circle all the vowels in these words. Notice that the number of vowels is often the same as the number of syllables in the word.

Example: potato

black   fishing   global   violin

goldfish	hotel	postcard	appendix
handicap	comprehend	phonograph	phenomenal
confiscate	daffodil	difficult	cafeteria
fantastic	umbrella	vitamin	ballot

EXERCISE 8. Consonants

The other important component of a syllable is the consonant. Circle all the consonants in these words.

Example: (p)o(t)a(t)o

fantastic	modification	club	skeptic
scarf	basket	microscope	confrontation
practical	maximum	bank	planet
imagine	trumpet	pumps	political

EXERCISE 9. Syllables

For these words, write the number of syllables in the space provided.

Example: potato _3_

calendar __	managers __	membership __	umbrella __
mechanical __	paragraph __	panic __	paper __
bishop __	disagree __	telegram __	calculator __
personal __	fundamental __	reporter __	particular __
percolator __	banana __	pilot __	basketball __

EXERCISE 10. Review

Circle the correct answer in these statements.

1. An accent is the result of *isolation / transfer from the native language.*

2. A dialect is the result of *isolation / transfer from the native language.*

3. The goal of accent modification is to *eliminate a person's accent / make a person's speech more understandable.*

4. A nonnative speaker of a language speaks a form of that language known as *interlanguage accent / dialect.*

5. "Relaxing the Muscles of the Face," Producing the Tone," and "Centering the Tone" are known as *primary speech elements / general adjustments in preparing to speak.*

6. Pitch and Rhythm are known as the *primary speech elements / secondary speech elements.*

7. The basic unit of speech is the *sound / word / syllable.*

8. In the word *democratic,* there are *6 / 4* vowels.

9. In the word *democratic,* there are *6 / 4* consonants.

10. In the word *democratic,* there are *6 / 4* syllables.

LESSON 3

Using Pitch in One- and Two-Syllable Words and Phrases

OBJECTIVE

In this lesson, you will learn about *pitch range*, *average pitch*, and the final *pitch fall*. You will also develop control of the *pitch* of your voice on useful one- and two-syllable words and phrases. Finally, you will learn that lip rounding is important to several common speech sounds.

PITCH RANGE AND AVERAGE PITCH

In Lesson 2, we learned that pitch is the most important element in American English speech. Therefore, appropriate pitch control is a very positive modification that a person can make. Let us begin with some useful concepts about this speech element.

In speaking American English, a person will vary the pitch of the voice. Because a range of pitch is used, it is necessary to determine what our potential range is. *Pitch range* is the series of tones that extends from a comfortable highest point to a comfortable lowest point. A sigh, as discussed in Exercise 1, is frequently used to determine a person's pitch range.

Within the total pitch range, every person has one pitch that is used most frequently. It is comfortable and sounds natural for that person. We call this *average pitch*. A person's average pitch will normally occur about five notes or steps above the lowest pitch in the pitch range. Average pitch is not exactly halfway between the highest and the lowest pitch in the pitch range. With the help of your teacher, you will easily be able to determine your average pitch.

EXERCISE 1. Developing an Awareness of Pitch and Pitch Range Using a Sigh

When speakers of American English see a beautiful picture, for example, they might produce a "sigh." The sigh is made by starting near the top of your comfortable pitch range and falling down to the bottom of your range. Frequently only a vowel is used on the downward pitch fall to produce a sigh. Practice by saying these vowels on a sigh.

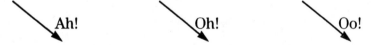

Ah!　　Oh!　　Oo!

CONTROLLING PITCH AT THE ENDS OF WORDS AND SENTENCES

American English requires a fall in pitch at the ends of words when said alone and at the end of sentences. The exercises in this lesson will help in gaining awareness and control of pitch. Remember to use a pitch range and an average pitch that are comfortable for you.

EXERCISE 2. "Monotone Speech"

Say the word *one* on your average pitch. Do not let the pitch of your voice change. Repeat *one* five times at the same pitch level. Repeat the word *two* five times without letting your pitch change. Pitch should not go up or down. Speech that has no pitch variation is called "monotone speech" and is not used by speakers of American English because it is not very interesting. We are using it to develop an awareness of our average pitch.

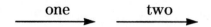

> **Pronunciation Note:** Remember to round your lips at the beginning of the word *one* because it is pronounced like *won*. Now say the word *two*. Once again, you will round your lips because the vowel is made with the lips rounded. Native speakers round their lips even when making the /t/ in *two*. Use a mirror to confirm that your lips are rounded.

EXERCISE 3. The Pitch Fall

As you say the word *one*, let your pitch fall (*Figure 3–1*). This is the American English <u>downward fall</u> that is used to end most sentences. Now repeat with the word *two*. The pitch fall indicates that the speaker has finished. Listen for the final pitch fall as used by speakers on television and in meetings and classes.

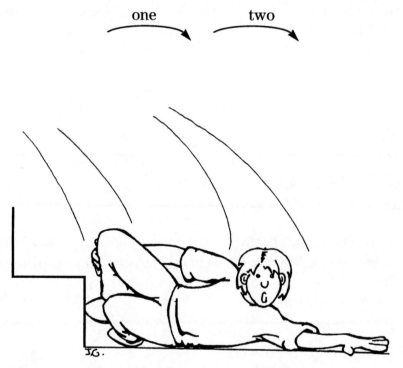

Figure 3–1. The pitch fall. A downward fall in pitch signals that the speaker is finished.

EXERCISE 4. Common Answers Said on the Pitch Fall

Practice these words by first saying each one on a sigh. Start on a pitch above your average pitch and fall down. You will see that each word is longer in duration when said on a sigh. Then practice these answers again, starting at your average pitch and falling. Each word will be shorter said this way than on a sigh.

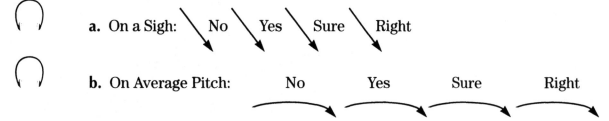

a. On a Sigh: No   Yes   Sure   Right

b. On Average Pitch: No   Yes   Sure   Right

c. Answer these questions asked by your instructor, using the words in Exercise 4b as answers.

Example: Instructor: Is that your book?
Student: Sure.

Is it raining today?

Are you going home after class?

Is your name Terry?

Do you feel sick?

Do you live in Chicago?

EXERCISE 5. Jumping on the Second Syllable

In this exercise, you will say *one* (the first syllable) on your average pitch. Then jump and fall in pitch on *two*. Do not glide from *one* to *two*, but jump up in pitch as demonstrated in *Figure 3–2*.

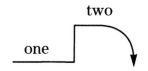

two

one

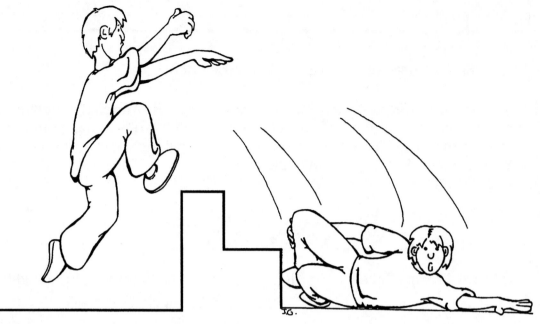

Figure 3–2. The pitch jump followed by the final fall. An upward jump in pitch precedes the fall.

EXERCISE 6. Practicing the Jump on the Second Syllable

Count as above. Then say these words and phrases.

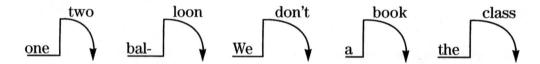

> **Pronunciation Note:** The words *a* and *the* are usually pronounced with the neutral vowel.

EXERCISE 7. Diagramming

Diagram these words and phrases as shown in Exercise 6. Then practice saying them.

today   She won't.   beside   return   I can't.   the desk   a dime

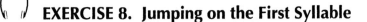

EXERCISE 8. Jumping on the First Syllable

In this exercise, we will count to *two* by starting (jumping) <u>above</u> average pitch on *one* and falling <u>below</u> average pitch for *two*. Use the downward fall as you say *two*. Remember to (1) use a pitch range that is comfortable for you, (2) round your lips, (3) use a constant loudness level, and (4) fall on the word *two*.

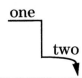

EXERCISE 9. Practicing the Jump on the First Syllable

Count as before and then say these words and phrases.

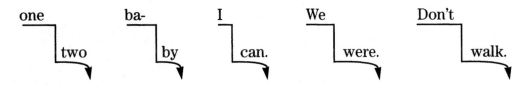

> **Pronunciation Note:** Speakers of American English frequently jump in pitch on negative words such as *don't, can't,* or *won't.* You can read more about the pitch jump on negative words in Lesson 8.

EXERCISE 10. Diagramming

Diagram these words and short sentences as demonstrated in Exercise 9. Then practice saying them.

over   under   Kay will.   author   scissors   city   John did.

EXERCISE 11. Choosing the Right Intonation

In these two-syllable words and phrases you will jump in pitch on either the <u>first</u> syllable or the <u>second</u> as shown in the examples. Decide which example—1 or 2—

each word or phrase fits, then write the corresponding example number in the space provided. You might have to ask a friend or look up the word in your dictionary (see Lesson 4) if you do not know where the pitch jump occurs.

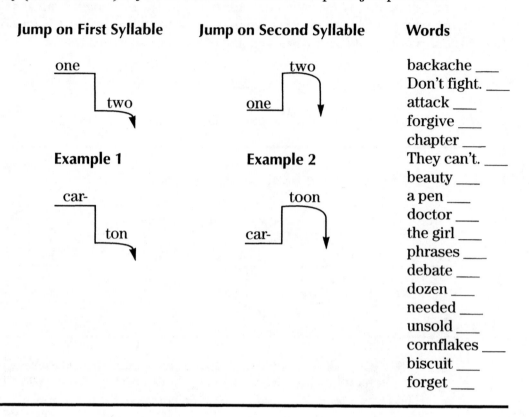

Jump on First Syllable	Jump on Second Syllable	Words

Example 1 | **Example 2**

Words

backache ___
Don't fight. ___
attack ___
forgive ___
chapter ___
They can't. ___
beauty ___
a pen ___
doctor ___
the girl ___
phrases ___
debate ___
dozen ___
needed ___
unsold ___
cornflakes ___
biscuit ___
forget ___

EXERCISE 12. Review Questions

Circle the correct answers for the following questions.

1. What do we call the pitch level that a person uses most frequently and comfortably in speaking?

   high pitch   low pitch   pitch range   average pitch

2. What do we call the series of tones, from high to low, that a person can produce?

   high pitch   low pitch   pitch range   average pitch

3. Is average pitch exactly half-way between the highest and the lowest pitch that a person can produce?

   Yes   No

4. When does the pitch fall occur most frequently in American English?

On every important word

On the last syllable

Never. Speakers use monotone speech.

5. A good way to identify your own pitch range is to:

Cry   Sing   Sigh   Cough

SOUND ADVICE

Some lessons in this text have a section called "sound advice" that will help in developing the skills needed for pronouncing the problem sounds in American English. Rather than focusing on how to make each of these sounds, an approach that is time consuming and difficult, we focus on the essential *process* used to produce each sound. If you understand and can use the process presented in "sound advice," your speech will become more understandable. The first process that we will explore is "lip rounding." You will quickly see that certain sounds can be improved greatly by making this simple adjustment along with appropriate use of pitch. Even in the exercises in "sound advice," you will be directed to use appropriate pitch. Remember, pitch is a <u>primary</u> speech element.

Lip Rounding

American English makes considerable use of lip rounding. For example, several vowels are always made with the lips rounded, as /uw/ in *glue*, /u/ in *good*, /aw/ in *caught*, and /o/ in *go*. Some important consonants are also rounded. The lips are never really spread as in a smile. When they are not rounded, they are relaxed. The best way to learn lip rounding is with the use of a small mirror. This process is extremely important and the time spent learning to round the lips is worth it. In American English the <u>corners of the mouth and the bottom lip</u> are more active than the <u>upper</u> lip. The upper lip may be generally relaxed while the bottom lip is rounded.

Lip Rounding and the /sh/, /zh/, /ch/, and /j/ Sounds

The /sh/ in *shop*, /zh/ in *vision*, /ch/ in *chop*, and /j/ in *jar* will sound better when rounded (Edwards, 1992). They are made with comfortable rounding (slight rounding). Once again, a mirror is useful in guiding your practice.

EXERCISE 13. Words for Practice

Round your lips for these sounds. Confirm this by using your mirror. On one syllable words, jump <u>and</u> fall in pitch on the same syllable. In two syllable words, jump in pitch on the syllable written in **boldface** type. If the jump occurs on the last syllable of a word, fall in pitch after the jump.

/sh/ words:	sure	shoot	shoe	short	chef
	show	**show**er	**su**gar	a**shamed**	**con**science
	cushion	**wash**rag	**work**shop	shock	**sha**dow
/zh/ words:	Asia	**fu**sion	**lei**sure	**trea**sure	**vi**sion
	Persian	**ver**sion	**mea**sure	**plea**sure	a**llu**sion
/ch/ words:	champ	child	church	choice	cheap
	sandwich	**chap**ter	Chi**nese**	**cul**ture	**chan**nel
	chair	**fu**ture	check	**kit**chen	charge
/j/ words:	gem	joke	**Ger**man	**gen**der	joint
	judge	germ	**gi**ant	Ja**pan**	**bud**get
	journal	**ju**nior	**ju**ry	**jel**ly	**jol**ly

No Lip Rounding

Many sounds in American English have no lip rounding. For these sounds, the lips are relaxed. One such sound is /l/ as in *let*. In addition to relaxed lips, for the /l/ at the beginning of syllables, the front of the tongue touches the gum ridge behind the upper teeth. Using your mirror, practice saying *lee-lee-lee* and *la-la-la* until you can make the /l/ sound appropriately.

EXERCISE 14. The Unrounded /l/: Words for Practice

Practice saying these words. Use your mirror to make sure that your lips remain unrounded on the /l/ sound.

leaf	lake	luck	look	late
lost	love	**la**bor	**li**mit	**li**ving
lion	**lu**nar	**so**lid	a**llow**	**ba**lance
dollar	co**llapse**	e**lect**	**co**llege	**lus**cious

LESSON 4

Using Pitch in Three-Syllable Words and Phrases

OBJECTIVE

In this lesson you will learn:

- ■ How to use pitch in words and phrases of three syllables;

- ■ How to pronounce contractions such as *I'm* and *they're*;

- ■ How to use your dictionary in accent modification;

- ■ How to start a personal *Pronunciation Notebook*; and

- ■ How to use airflow in producing several common speech sounds.

INTRODUCTION

The principles that you studied in Lessons 2 and 3 will be expanded in this lesson. In words and phrases of three syllables, it is possible to place the pitch jump on any one of the three syllables as will be shown in these exercises.

EXERCISE 1. Counting to Three

Start above your average pitch on *one* and step down to your average pitch for *two*. For *three* use the downward fall. Try to keep the same loudness level on each number. Remember: jump on *one*, step down on *two*, and fall on *three* (*Figure 4–1*).

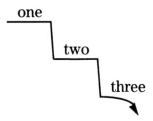

EXERCISE 2. Practicing Words and Phrases

Count as above. Then practice these words and phrases. Continue to jump on the first syllable, step down on the second syllable, and fall in pitch on the third syllable.

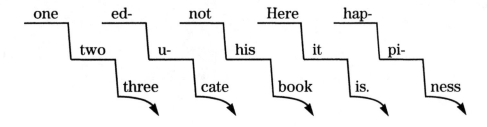

EXERCISE 3. Diagramming

Diagram these words and phrases as shown in Exercise 2. Then practice saying them.

quality   microphone   visitor   Don't tell me.   Who is it?

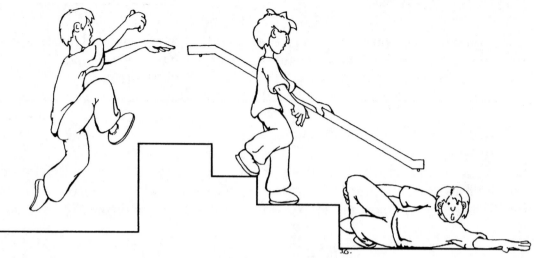

Figure 4–1. Jump, Step, Fall. After the pitch jump, speakers of American English step down in pitch and then let their pitch fall.

EXERCISE 4. A Three-Syllable Variation

Now vary the pitch by starting on your average pitch for *one*, jumping up to *two*, and then falling down on *three*. The final syllable will be longer because of the pitch fall.

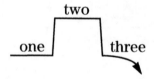

EXERCISE 5. Practicing Words and Phrases

Count as above, then say these words and phrases.

EXERCISE 6. Diagramming

Diagram these words and phrases as shown in Exercise 5. Then practice saying them.

I think so.   the bookstore   Believe me.   promoting

develop   together

EXERCISE 7. Choosing the Right Intonation.

Here are some words that fit one of the two variations that you have learned in this lesson. Decide which pattern each word or phrase fits — <u>Example 1</u> or <u>Example 2</u>, and write the corresponding number — 1 or 2 — in the space provided.

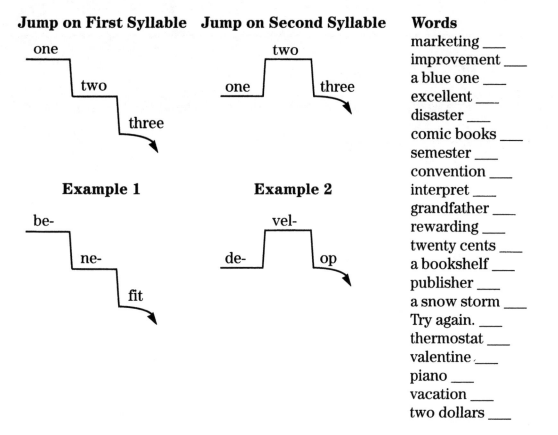

Jump on First Syllable	Jump on Second Syllable
Example 1	Example 2

Words

marketing ___
improvement ___
a blue one ___
excellent ___
disaster ___
comic books ___
semester ___
convention ___
interpret ___
grandfather ___
rewarding ___
twenty cents ___
a bookshelf ___
publisher ___
a snow storm ___
Try again. ___
thermostat ___
valentine ___
piano ___
vacation ___
two dollars ___

EXERCISE 8. Jumping and Falling on the Last Syllable

For this exercise, maintain your average pitch for <u>both</u> *one* and *two*. In other words, "walk" through the first two syllables without changing your average pitch as demonstrated in *Figure 4-2*. Then jump <u>and</u> fall in pitch on *three*. This means that when you jump on *three*, you must also lengthen the vowel so you will have time to let your pitch fall on the final syllable.

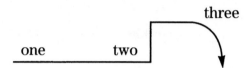

EXERCISE 9. Phrases For Practice

Count as above. Then practice these phrases.

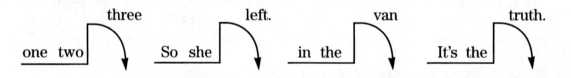

Exercise 10. Diagramming

Diagram these words and phrases as in Exercise 9. Then practice saying them.

on the floor   in the car   But we won't.   It's a girl.

I forgot   recommend   underneath

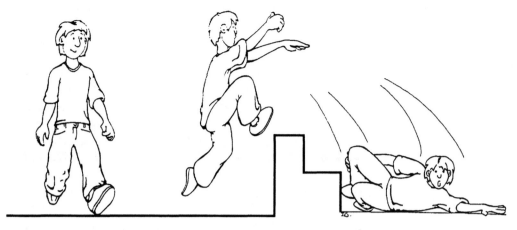

Figure 4–2. Walk, Jump, Fall. Walk without changing average pitch, then jump and fall.

EXERCISE 11. Choosing the Right Intonation

Here are some words that fit one of the three variations that you have learned in this lesson. Decide which pattern each word or phrase fits — Example 1, Example 2, or Example 3 — and write the corresponding number — 1, 2, or 3— in the space provided.

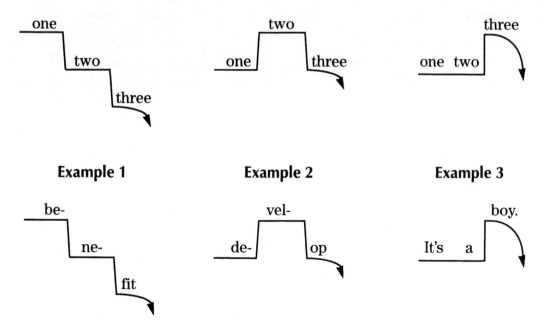

Jump on First Syllable   **Jump on Second Syllable**   **Jump on Third Syllable**

one
    two
        three

    two
one   three

    three
one two

Example 1   **Example 2**   **Example 3**

be-
   ne-
     fit

   vel-
de-   op

   boy.
It's a

Words

on the phone ___	misinform ___	chewing gum ___	condition ___
performance ___	digestion ___	sandwiches ___	comprehend ___
dialect ___	They're not home. ___	sunflower ___	understand ___
beautiful ___	He's just ten. ___	library ___	in the park ___

EXERCISE 12. Pronouncing Contractions

Speakers of American English prefer to use contractions rather than more formal speech without contractions. In a contraction, there is a loss of a syllable, so that *I am* (two syllables) becomes *I'm* (one syllable). Practice pronouncing these uncontracted and contracted forms.

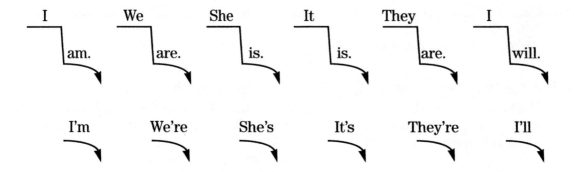

> ***Pronunciation Note:*** Contractions are not used as complete sentences. When asked, *Who's ready?*, the answer is, *I am*, not *I'm*. Use the contraction when another word follows, as in *I'm ready.*

EXERCISE 13. Practicing Contractions

In the space provided, answer each of these questions with a contraction and the appropriate word from the list of choices. On those answers requiring a *yes*, jump up and fall on the word *Yes*. Then complete the rest of the response. Next, your teacher will ask these questions. Answer using what you have written.

List of Choices: *fine, done, sure, ready, here, home, wait*

Example: Teacher: Are you ready?   Student: **Yes**. I'm **rea**dy.

Teacher:	Are they done?	Student:	Yes. _____
	Is she ready?		Yes. _____
	Where are you?		_____
	Will they wait?		Yes. _____
	How is he today?		_____
	Where is Mary?		_____
	Are you done?		Yes. _____
	Is John ready?		Yes. _____
	How is Mary?		_____
	Will you wait?		Yes. _____
	Are you sure?		Yes. _____

EXERCISE 14. Pronouncing Your Name

Your name is very special. However, the pronunciation of names is a common source of misunderstanding. As our goal in accent modification is understanding, you might be able to use one of the patterns provided in this lesson when people ask you your name. We will learn to pronounce your first name (or the name that you use) so that speakers of American English will understand.

1. Ask your teacher for help in deciding how to say your first name, or the name you wish to use. Where will you jump in pitch? How will you step down? How will you fall at the end? Now diagram your first name here.

2. Answer this question asked by your teacher. Say only your name as you diagrammed it in #1.

   Teacher: What's your name? *(Say your name as diagrammed in #1.)*

3. Now answer the question with a more complete response: *My name's* (insert your name here). The words *My name's* should be spoken on your average pitch level.

   Example: Teacher: What's your name?

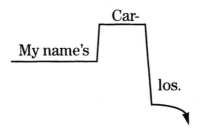

(Substitute your name as diagrammed in #1.)

4. Now practice <u>both</u> answers to the question, "What's your name?"

    a. Say your name. Then say the complete pattern.
        Example: Teacher: What's your name?
                    Student: Carlos. My name's Carlos.

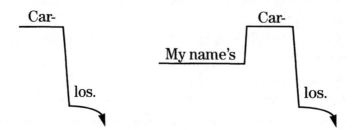

    b. Now add your last name. Continue stepping down after you've said your first name.
        Example: Teacher: What's your name?
                    Student: Carlos. My name's Carlos. Carlos Gómez.

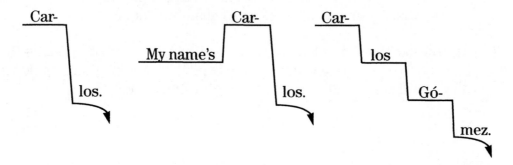

5. On a map of the world, locate your home country. Then introduce yourself as in the example. Jump in pitch on your first name <u>and</u> on the name of your country. The pitch jumps are written in **boldface** type in the example.

    Example: Student: My name's **Car**los. **Car**los Gómez. I'm from **Mex**ico.

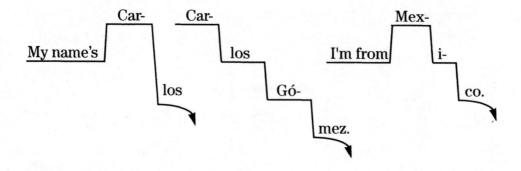

EXERCISE 15. Pronouncing Names

Here are some common names that you might need to pronounce. Diagram them in the space provided. Jump in pitch on the syllables in **boldface** type.

Janette   Anita   **David**   Alexander

EXERCISE 16. Practicing Names That You Know

Ask at least three of your American English-speaking friends to say their first names. Listen to the intonation that they use. Diagram the names in the space provided.

USING YOUR DICTIONARY TO DETERMINE WHERE TO JUMP IN PITCH

Your dictionary can help you decide where to jump in pitch. Look at the pronunciation of the words listed below as they might appear in a standard American English dictionary. A stress mark like this ' tells you to jump in pitch on this syllable. Some dictionaries will place the stress mark *before* the syllable to be stressed; others place it *after* the stressed syllable. Once you determine how your dictionary marks "jump" syllables, then step down on each syllable after that, and fall in pitch on the last syllable. In longer words some dictionaries have a lighter mark on another syllable. Use the darker mark in determining where to jump.

Example:

WORD	DICTIONARY PRONUNCIATION	DIAGRAM
develop	di vel' əp	
recommend	rek ə mend'	
benefit	ben' ə fit	

Note. Random House Webster's College Dictionary (1991) was used for the words in these examples.

EXERCISE 17. Using Your Dictionary

Use your dictionary to help you pronounce the following words. Then diagram them as in the examples.

marshmallow   disappoint

discover   calendar

indirect   disagree

contagious   educate

attention   revenue

EXERCISE 18. Starting your Pronunciation Notebook

Using the pages in Appendix C of this text, or in a notebook that you have called your "Pronunciation Notebook for Accent Modification," begin a section titled "Words I Use Every day." Then write four words of no more than three syllables that you use at work, in class, or with your English-speaking friends. Some examples might be *develop, accounting, Saturday, designer, educate, deposit,* or *physics*. Organize your words into three columns as in the example. In the first space, write the word. Then copy the way the word is "pronounced" in the dictionary. Finally, diagram the word. Once the words have been checked by your instructor, practice saying them until they are understandable.

WORDS I USE EVERY DAY

WORD	DICTIONARY	DIAGRAM
develop	di vel' əp	

SOUND ADVICE

Airflow

All languages depend on airflow from the lungs for speech. The air stream coming from the lungs makes the vocal cords vibrate and causes the air in the throat, mouth, and nose to resonate. We speak on expired air. However, languages use airflow in different ways to produce sounds. For example, some sounds, such as /h/, /s/, /f/, and /v/ require *continuous* airflow during the time the sound is being produced. At other times a sound may interrupt the airflow for a moment before it is released again. Some sounds that are made with *interrupted* airflow are /p/, /b/, /t/, /d/, /k/, and /g/. See *Figure 4–3*.

Continuous Airflow for /h/, /s/, /f/, and /v/

These important sounds require airflow. Many languages have similar airflow on these sounds.

AIRFLOW

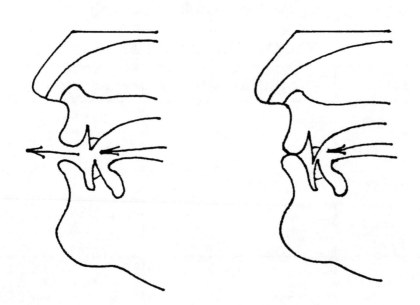

CONTINUOUS   INTERRUPTED

Figure 4–3. The two kinds of airflow. Sounds may be produced with continuous or interrupted airflow.

EXERCISE 19. Words for Practice

Try to feel the airflow as you say these words. The syllable receiving the pitch jump is written in **boldface** type.

/h/:	home	health	hope	**ha**mmer	house
	re**hearse**	**han**dle	hand	hall	hat
	hamburger	**ho**liday	happy	in**her**it	head
/s/:	see	sat	seat	safe	set
	Sunday	**so**da	**sub**way	**some**body	**Sat**urday
/f/:	feel	face	fine	phone	food
	final	**fun**ny	**pho**nograph	foun**da**tion	fi**nan**cial
/v/:	verb	van	voice	**vine**yard	**va**lue
	vitamin	ad**vice**	**bea**ver	Bev	**nev**er
	wave	a**vai**lable	a**bu**sive	**car**nival	be**lieve**

Continuous Airflow on Voiceless /th/ and Voiced /TH/

If you use a /t/ or a /d/ instead of these sounds, you are not producing them with sufficient airflow. When you make these sounds correctly, there should be a continuous flow of air. You might find it useful to make /s/, and while the air is flowing, make the /th/ sound. This same procedure can be used to turn /z/ into a /TH/.

Examples of /th/: theme, thick, thief, thumb, thought, thin, thing, thanks

Examples of /TH/: this, those, that, their, then, the, though

EXERCISE 20. Practice with the Voiceless /th/

> ***Pronunciation Note:*** If you use /s/ or /z/ instead of /th/ or /TH/, the problem is not with airflow, but with tongue placement. The tongue is back too far from the teeth and should be moved forward to make light contact with the upper *and* lower teeth.

Touch your teeth lightly with your tongue. Be sure there is airflow. Continue to jump in pitch on the syllable in **boldface** type.

theme	**thea**ter	**theo**ry
thing	third	**thir**sty
Thursday	**thir**ty	thir**teen**
with	both	math
teeth	mouth	south
north	truth	health
length	**se**venth	month
something	north**west**	**birth**day
faithful	with**in**	**au**thor

Exercise 21. Practice with the Voiced /TH/

With the same tongue position and airflow as for /th/, turn your voice on to produce /TH/.

then	these	they
them	though	there
either	**lea**ther	**fa**ther
mother	**bro**ther	**clo**thing
weather	**o**ther	an**o**ther
their	the	that
those	to**ge**ther	this

Interrupted Airflow on /p/ and /b/

Few students of American English have difficulty with /t/, /d/, /k/, or /g/, even though they are made with interrupted airflow. The /p/ and /b/ sounds, however, may require a little extra concentration so that the airflow is clearly interrupted. Otherwise, a listener may hear /f/ for /p/ and /v/ for /b/.

EXERCISE 22. Practice with /p/

In saying these words, make sure that the airflow is blocked for a moment. This action actually puts a very short pause into your speech. The syllable in two syllable words, written in **boldface** type, should receive the pitch jump.

pep	pop	part
pepper	**po**pping	puff
supper	slope	help
stopping	per**fume**	flip

Exercise 23. Practice with /b/

In addition to interrupted airflow, words with /b/ require voice. In words of more than one syllable, the pitch jump will occur on the syllable written in **boldface** type.

bib	Bob	**tab**let
bumper	be**have**	a**bove**
label	**ba**by	**ver**bal
brave	vi**bra**tion	**be**verage
sobbing	buy	rib
ribbon	ob**serve**	**bath**tub

LESSON 5

Using Pitch In Phrases And Sentences

OBJECTIVE

In Lesson 4, you learned to control three levels of pitch, as in "Where is John?" In this lesson, you will learn how to use up to five pitch levels, and how to say several syllables or words on the same pitch level. You will also add more important words to your personal *Pronunciation Notebook*.

Things to Remember:

■ Daily practice is necessary to obtain control of pitch.

■ Speakers of American English use pitch more than the other speech elements.

■ Use the pitch jump instead of loudness for syllable, word, or sentence emphasis (stress).

■ Speakers of American English jump up or step down when changing from one pitch level to another.

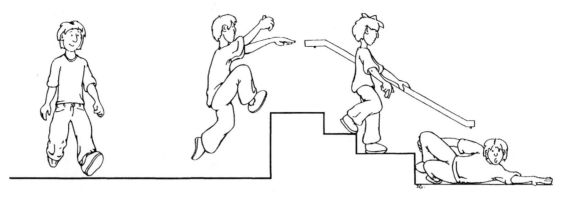

Figure 5–1. *Walk, Jump, Step, Fall:* Standard Intonation.

STANDARD INTONATION: *WALK, JUMP, STEP, FALL*

Speakers of American English *walk* on their average pitch to an important word in a phrase or sentence. Then they *jump* in pitch on the prominent syllable of that word (Stern, 1991). Next, they *step down* in pitch on each syllable to the end of the sentence, and *fall* in pitch on the last syllable. This is known as *standard intonation* and is easily remembered in the phrase: *walk, jump, step, fall (Figure 5-1)*. Students must decide where to jump, how high to jump, how to step down on each syllable following the jump, and how to make the steps small enough so that there is sufficient pitch left for the fall at the end of the sentence. In American English, the pitch fall is used at the end of the sentence to signal completion of the thought. It tells your listener that you are finished.

COMMON QUESTIONS THAT STUDENTS ASK

Where does the pitch jump occur in the sentence?

Many speakers prefer to place it *early* in the sentence. The pitch jump is always connected to the meaning of the sentence: the most meaningful word in the sentence has the highest pitch. We will return to this important topic in a later lesson.

Can I use too many pitch jumps in a sentence?

Yes. American English speakers usually limit the number of pitch jumps in a sentence to one or two. If a sentence has too many jumps, it is confusing to listeners and has irregular rhythm.

What happens *before* the pitch jump?

If the pitch jump does not occur on the first syllable of the phrase or sentence, speakers of American English usually walk on their average pitch to the place where the pitch jump will occur. This means that average pitch is maintained almost in a monotone until the jump. Walking our pitch in this manner helps to focus the listener's attention on the most important part of what we say.

What happens *after* the pitch jump?

Speakers of American English step down on every syllable after the pitch jump. A sentence with more syllables will have more steps which will be smaller than in a sentence with fewer syllables. Students must learn to control both the number and size of the steps in the sentence.

What happens to pitch at the end of a sentence?

Typically, the pitch at the end of an American English sentence falls. This means that the size of the step from the pitch jump to the last syllable must allow for the final fall. If the steps have been too large, there will not be sufficient pitch range left for the fall. Therefore, the *walk, jump, step, fall* must be coordinated.

COMMON MISTAKES IN USING *WALK, JUMP, STEP, FALL*

- ■ Not jumping at all in a sentence
- ■ Jumping too many times in a sentence
- ■ Jumping on an unimportant word
- ■ Jumping on the wrong syllable of the word selected for the jump
- ■ Not stepping down on every syllable following the pitch jump
- ■ Using pitch steps that are too large
- ■ Not falling in pitch on the last syllable

WORKING WITH SEVERAL PITCH LEVELS

One of the values of this approach to accent modification is that students do not have to memorize many sentence patterns. All of the variations of standard *walk, jump, step, fall* intonation are determined by the position of the pitch jump in the sentence. Once the pitch jump has occurred, the step down and fall parts of the sentence are predictable, based on the number of syllables from the pitch jump to the end of the sentence.

The following activities will help you to develop control in the use of walk, jump, step, fall. Note that the jump in pitch is specified for you. Do not jump in pitch on any other word or syllable.

EXERCISE 1. Determining the Number of Syllables

Draw a line between all the syllables as shown in the example. Then count the number of syllables in the entire sentence and write the number in the space provided. Finally, count the number of syllables from the pitch jump (the syllable in **boldface** type) to the end of the sentence, and write that number on the next line. Remember that the steps and fall will occur on the syllables <u>following</u> the pitch jump.

Example: The/ **news**/pa/per/ has/ ma/ny/ ar/ti/cles/ on/ e/co/no/mics./ <u>15</u> Syllables <u>13</u>

My **birth**day is in September. _____ _____

One of the students is from Mexico. _____ _____

We re**ceived** a telegram on Saturday. _____ _____

My **par**ents are going on vacation in August. _____ _____

We ob**served** Jupiter through a telescope. _____ _____

The **se**nators approved the legislation. _____ _____

Modifying your accent is important. _____ _____

The **te**lephone was invented by Alexander Graham Bell. _____ _____

EXERCISE 2. Jumping on the Second Syllable

In this exercise, the pitch jump occurs on the second syllable (*two*) with step down on *three* and *four*, and the fall on *five*. Repeat it until you can hear your voice do what it is supposed to do. Do not increase loudness on the pitch jump.

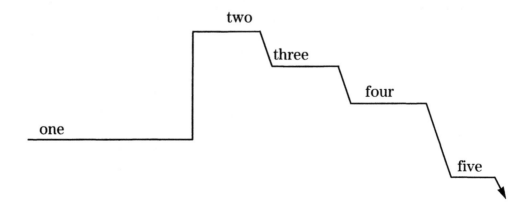

> ***Pronunciation Note:*** In stepping down in pitch from the pitch jump, the critical step is the syllable immediately following the jump. In this example, the *three* is critical. If your pitch steps are too large, your pitch range will not be sufficient for the following steps, and you will not be able to fall appropriately on the last syllable. The solution to this problem is to make sure that your first pitch step down is small enough to allow for the fall in pitch at the end of the sentence. Take small steps down after the jump, starting with the first syllable *after* the jump.

EXERCISE 3. Sentences for Practice

Practice the sentences using the example from Exercise 1. Then present the story. Jump in pitch on the word or syllable in **boldface** type. For the moment, ignore the asterisk (*) before the last sentence.

The **boys** drove away.

I **don't** want to go.

She **left** after school.

It's **ea**sy to do.

*The **cat** likes to play.

> **Story:** "The **Great** Fishing Trip"
> The **kids** went fishing.
> They **caught** lots of fish.
> Dad **cooked** all the fish.
> Their **din**ner was fine.

EXERCISE 4. Jumping on the Third Syllable

In this exercise, walk your average pitch through *one* and *two*. The pitch jump occurs on *three* with the step down on *four*, and fall on *five*. Continue your practice until you have complete control of each number.

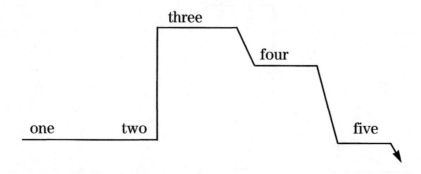

EXERCISE 5. Sentences for Practice

Practice these sentences using the example from Exercise 4. Then tell the story.

We have **three** of them.

We are **al**most done.

He is **ne**ver late.

John is **lear**ning fast.

*She is **ve**ry smart.

> **Story:** "It's the **Class** I Love"
> I have **four** classes.
> They are **all** quite good.
> I like **math** the best.
> It is **real**ly fun.

EXERCISE 6. A Longer Sentence Variation

This example is similar to the one in Exercises 4 and 5. Walk your pitch on *one* and *two*, jump on *three*, step down on *four* and *five*, and fall on *six*.

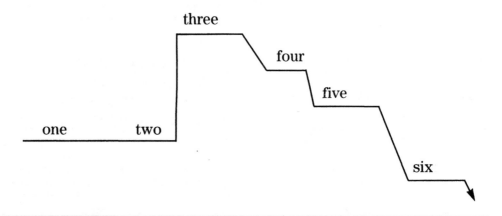

EXERCISE 7. Sentences for Practice

Practice these sentences using the example from Exercise 6.

It was **time** to go home.

We can **play** until six.

I was **wal**king the dog.

She did **not** want to go.

*I have **time** to relax.

> **Story:** "When the **Wea**ther is Bad"
> I was **driving** to work.
> It was **rain**ing quite hard.
> I could **not** see the road.
> So I **turned** on the lights.

EXERCISE 8. Jumping Toward the End of a Sentence

In this exercise, walk your pitch through numbers *one* to *four* because they are all said on the <u>same</u> pitch level. The jump occurs on *five* and the step down <u>and</u> fall on *six*.

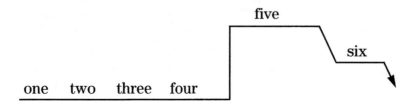

EXERCISE 9. Sentences for Practice

Practice these sentences using the form shown in Exercise 8 as your guide.

The girl and boy **love** it.

The children are **hap**py.

Mary Brown is **mo**ving.

I have an ap**point**ment.

*We'll try to **help** you.

> **Story:** "When You Need Ad**vis**ing"
> My schedule is **aw**ful.
> The homework is **too** hard.
> My classes are **bor**ing.
> I need my ad**vis**or.

> ***Pronunciation Note:*** In the sentences in Exercise 9, other possibilities for the pitch jump exist. You will learn about *special emphasis* in Lesson 12.

EXERCISE 10. A Useful Variation with the Jump on the First Syllable

The sentence form in this activity is useful for some later lessons that we will have. The jump occurs on *one* with the step down on every syllable thereafter to the fall in pitch on *five*.

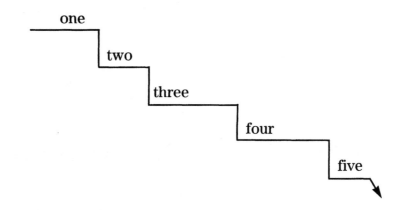

EXERCISE 11. Sentences for Practice

These sentences make use of the form shown in Exercise 10. Practice each sentence carefully, making sure that you step down on each syllable after the pitch jump. Remember to fall on the last syllable of each sentence.

Where does Tom Jones live?

How are you feeling?

How much is it worth?

They found the answer.

Wait just a minute.

*__When__ did you arrive?

> **Story:** "**Who** Bought the Last Book?"
> **Jane** bought the last book.
> **Where** did she get it ?
> **When** did she buy it?
> **I** think I'll ask her.

> ***Pronunciation Note:*** Notice that the questions in this exercise have the pitch fall at the end. As we will see in Lesson 7, questions of this type are asked with falling pitch.

EXERCISE 12. What's Your Name?

Now repeat Exercise 14 from Lesson 4, as shown in this example.

Example: Student 1: What's your name?

Student 2: Carlos. My name's Carlos.

EXERCISE 13. Diagramming Sentences

Diagram all the sentences in Exercises 3, 5, 7, 9, and 11 marked with an asterisk (*).

The cat likes to play.

I have time to relax.

She is very smart.

We'll try to help you.

When did you arrive?

EXERCISE 14. Stories for Practice

In these two stories you will review the forms studied in this lesson. Walk to the syllable in **boldface** type and jump on that syllable. Step down in pitch on each syllable that follows. Use the pitch fall on the last syllable.

Story 1: **NO** TIME FOR LUNCH	**Story 2**: **BAD** WEATHER
It was **twelve** o'clock.	The **wea**ther is bad.
I was **rea**dy for lunch.	It's **very** windy.
Who would go with me?	There's **ice** on the streets.
My friends had ap**point**ments.	**Dri**ving is risky.
I **went** out alone.	I'd like to be **home** now.
	I **can't** wait for spring.

EXERCISE 15. Adding More Useful Words to Your *Pronunciation Notebook*

In Lesson 4, you wrote some words that you use every day that contained three syllables or less. Continue your list, using Appendix C, by writing down at least five words or phrases that you use every day. Some examples might be *mechanical engineering, education, university*, and *business administration*. Diagram each. Once they have been checked by your instructor, practice until they are understandable. Add words or phrases to your *Pronunciation Notebook* regularly.

EXERCISE 16. Review

Circle the correct answer in these statements.

1. The most important speech element for American English is *loudness / pitch*.

2. The part of a phrase or sentence occurring before the pitch jump is said on *a sigh / average pitch*.

3. The word selected for the pitch jump will usually occur *early / late* in sentences.

4. Meaning determines where the *high / low* pitch jump will occur.

5. Jump *many times / only one time* in short sentences.

6. At the end of most American English sentences, pitch *falls / jumps*.

7. A common mistake that students make is *stepping down on every syllable following the pitch jump / not stepping down*.

8. The sentence, *My Pro**nun**ciation Notebook contains important words*, has *14 / 15* syllables.

9. In the sentence, *My Pro**nun**ciation Notebook contains important words*, we *walk / fall* on the first two syllables.

10. There are *11 / 12* syllable steps <u>following</u> the pitch jump in the sentence in questions 8 and 9.

SOUND ADVICE

Lip Rounding: Slight and Tight

There are two kinds of lip rounding in American English which differ primarily in degree. For some sounds, the lips are slightly or comfortably rounded (*Figure 5–2*), whereas for other sounds, the lips are tightly rounded and protruded with considerable effort (*Figure 5–3*). The first type of rounding is more open, but for the second type of rounding, the lips are close together. In addition to the rounded sounds studied in Lesson 3 (/sh/, /zh/, /ch/ and /j/), the American English /r/ sound will also sound better if it is made with lip rounding. Make sure that the tongue does not touch the front teeth. By rounding the lips, it is easier to make this sound.

Lip Rounding and the /r/ Sound

The American English /r/ sound is one of the most difficult to produce. The lips are slightly rounded with sufficient space between the upper and lower lips to

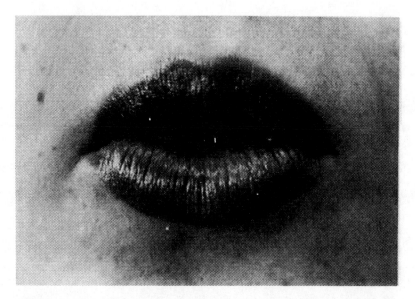

Figure 5–2. Slight lip rounding. The lips are comfortably rounded /r/.

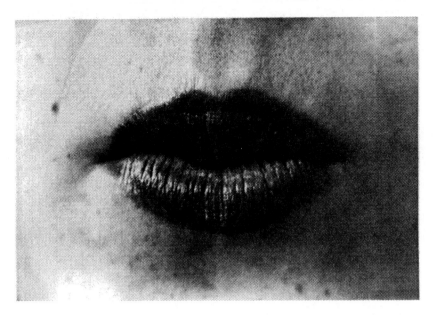

Figure 5–3. Tight lip rounding. The lips are tightly rounded for /w/.

insert a ballpoint pen! You will not be able to make an acceptable /r/ sound unless you learn to round your lips in this manner. Use your mirror to check your production of the /r/ in these words.

EXERCISE 17. The Rounded /r/: Words for Practice

Say the following words of one or two syllables. Be sure to jump <u>and</u> fall on the one syllable words. On the two syllable words, jump on the appropriate syllable (in **boldface**).

a. **Rounded /r/ with a Rounded Vowel.** These /r/ words should be easier to pronounce because the lips are rounded for the vowel that follows the /r/. Use your mirror.

robe	roof	rou**tine**	**ru**by	**ro**tate
arrow	road	rule	rope	ro**mance**
row	room	**ro**bot	**ru**in	rose

b. **Rounded /r/ with Other Vowels.** These /r/ words may be more difficult to pronounce because they occur with vowels that are not rounded.

ride	reach	race	**ra**bbit	**ra**cket	right

rare	**ra**dio	**rea**son	**ro**bber	re**volve**	**ri**pple
re**mark**	**rea**der	re**turn**	**ri**pen	red	**res**cue

c. **Rounded /r/ with All Kinds of Vowels.** All of theses words have the same /r/ sound as the word at the top of each list.

AIR	ARE	OR	HER	EAR
care	far	corn	were	near
hair	hard	warm	**thirs**ty	cheer
bear	car	your	worms	here
there	star	worn	fur	clear
fair	**car**bon	war	**ear**ly	ap**pear**
share	large	four	work	**spir**it
prayer	**par**don	score	word	fear
very	**tar**get	**cor**ner	bird	ca**shier**
Terry	barn	**or**der	church	deer
error	charge	ward	**eff**ort	**ear**ring

Lip Rounding and the /w/ Sound

The American English /w/ should be made with strong lip rounding. The lips are close together with no space between for a ballpoint pen! Focus on the lips for producing this sound rather than on the position of the tongue in the back of the mouth. If you concentrate on the lips, you will eliminate the tendency of some speakers to use a /gw/ combination for this sound. Use your mirror to confirm that you are producing this sound correctly. Do not spread your lips. Remember that the lips are either relaxed or rounded during American English speech. Spreading the lips (as for a smile or many sounds in other languages) causes some speech sounds to change. If the lips are spread during the /r/ sound, you will tend to produce the flap or trilled /r/ found in many languages, but not in American English. If you spread your lips during /w/, you will produce a sound more like a /v/ than a /w/. Facial muscles cannot be relaxed if the lips are spread.

Exercise 18. The Rounded /w/: Words for Practice

The following words contain the /w/ sound. Use your mirror to confirm that your lips are round. Jump and fall on the one syllable words; on the two syllable words, jump on the syllable that is written in **boldface** type.

a. Rounded /w/ with a Rounded Vowel. The following words which contain the /w/ sound should be easier to pronounce because the vowel that follows /w/ is also rounded.

wood	word	worth	**wor**ker	won't	**wo**man
homework	**wood**work	wool	a**woke**	world	**net**work

b. Rounded /w/ with Other Vowels. In the following words the /w/ occurs with vowel sounds that are not rounded. Use your mirror to confirm that you lips are rounded for the /w/.

re**ward**	**weal**thy	be**ware**	wage	wave	**win**dow
weigh	weave	**won**der	**wa**ter	were	will
wife	**wea**ther	a**way**	which	what	when
why	wheat	where	want	wish	weed

LESSON 6

Useful Phrases and Sentences

OBJECTIVE

In this lesson, you will use standard *walk, jump, step, fall* intonation in common phrases and sentences. We will also practice sounds requiring continuous and interrupted airflow, and lip rounding in sentences.

COMMON PHRASES

Perhaps you have not felt comfortable putting the principles you have learned into your speech outside of class. When we are given new procedures, we frequently do not know how to begin to implement them. In this lesson, you are given some very practical phrases and sentences that you can use every day with appropriate *walk, jump, step, fall* intonation. They provide us with a perfect place to start.

EXERCISE 1. Phrases and Sentences to Diagram and Practice

Diagram each phrase or sentence in the space provided. Then practice saying each, making sure the pitch of your voice follows the diagram. In practicing the following phrases and sentences, jump in pitch on the syllable or word written in **boldface** type.

1. Good **mor**ning.

2. **How** are you today?

3. I'm **just** fine.

4. **Thank** you.

5. July 4, 1776 (**July** fourth, seventeen seventy-six)

6. **What** time is it?

7. It's **lunch** time.

8. It's el**e**ven thirty. (11:30 AM)

9. **What's** your address?

10. 123 45th Street (**one**-twenty-three, forty-fifth street)

11. **Excuse** me.

12. I'm **sorry**.

13. It's **my** fault.

14. **Here** it is.

15. **How** much is it?

16. $19.50 (**Nine**teen dollars and fifty cents; **Nine**teen-fifty)

17. I **think** I'll look around.

18. I can **do** it.

19. I **can't** do it.

20. **Please** speak more slowly.

21. **What's** your telephone number?

22. My number is **five**-five-five, one-two-three-four (**5**55-1234).

23. **I'll** call later.

24. Walk, **jump**, step, fall

25. **a**ccent modification

Pronunciation Note: Telephone numbers, dates, addresses, time, and money usually require that the pitch jump occur at the beginning of the phrase, followed by the step down and fall at the end. In a seven-digit telephone number, jump in pitch on the first number. Then step down on each number that follows. Fall on the last number, for example, *555-1234* (*five-five-five, one-two-three-four*). Dates, addresses, time, and money phrases may follow the same pattern. The date, *December 4, 1910,* for example, is said *December fourth, nineteen-ten,* and the address, *123 45th Street,* is said *one-twenty-three, forty-fifth street.* Monetary values such as *$21.65,* are said *twenty-one dollars and sixty-five cents, or* simply, *twenty-one, sixty-five.* In each of these cases, a pattern that will always work is to jump in pitch at the beginning, step down on each following syllable, and fall on the last syllable.

EXERCISE 2. Phrases and Sentences for Substitution Drill

Practice the sentences in this exercise as written. Then substitute the new words into each as shown in the example. Your teacher will provide additional words for practice. Continue to use appropriate pitch control for these slightly longer phrases and sentences.

Example: Student: I **have** to call Professor Walker.
Teacher: write
Student: I **have** to write Professor Walker.
Teacher: him
Student: I **have** to write him.

1. I'm **sure** I can help you.
positive
them
fix

2. **Which** one do you want?
   they
   need
   boxes

3. **Please** show me some others.
   give
   them
   the
   papers.

4. It costs **Eigh**ty-five, ninety-five. ($85.95)
   They
   $17.88 (**se**venteen, eighty-eight)
   The shoes
   $34.15 (**thir**ty-four, fifteen)

5. I **want** a pair of shoes.
   They
   gloves.
   need

6. **What** kind of job do you want?
   car
   they
   drive?

7. I have an ap**point**ment.
   We
   want
   a**part**ment.

8. My **friend** gave me her telephone number.
   Our
   us
   social security
   teacher

9. That's **all** I have.
   want
   It's
   everything

10. She lives at **6**25 Elm Street. (**six**, twenty-five)
    400 (**four**-hundred)
    Park
    works
    Avenue

11. I'd **like** to apply for a job.
    We'd
    credit card.
    scholarship.

12. They left on No**vem**ber 5, 1965. (No**vem**ber fifth, nineteen sixty-five)
    We
    De**cem**ber 24 (De**cem**ber twenty-fourth)
    1972 (nineteen seventy-two)
    came

13. **Where** are my glasses?
    books?
    those
    What

14. She's **not** here today.
    now.
    Mary's
    in school

15. I'm an ac**coun**tant.
    He's
    (a) **law**yer.
    She's

EXERCISE 3. What Should You Say?

Answer these questions with appropriate phrases and sentences from Exercises 1 and 2. The first 14 questions are answered from Exercise 1 and the last four questions are best answered from Exercise 2.

Example: What should you say when . . .
  you go to ask for a job? *I'd **like** to apply for a job.*

What should you say when . . .

1. you step on someone's foot?

2. someone is speaking too fast?

3. you meet someone at 8 AM?

4. someone asks how you are?

5. you don't know the time?

6. you make a mistake?

7. it's 12 o'clock noon?

8. someone asks for your telephone number?

9. someone asks what class you are taking?

10. someone asks for your address?

11. your teacher asks you to describe American English intonation?

12. someone asks the time?

13. someone asks the date? (month, day, year)

14. you want to know what something costs?

15. you can help someone?

16. you have no more pencils to give your friend?

17. you lose your glasses?

18. you want to see some other examples?

DIALOGS FOR PRACTICE

The following dialogs are based on the phrases and sentences that you have already learned. Practice them until they are familiar and understandable.

Dialog 1: AN AP**POINT**MENT FOR A JOB

1st person: Good **mor**ning.

2nd person: I **need** to see Mr. Smith. I have an ap**point**ment.

1st person: I'm **sorry**. He's **sick**. He's **not** here today.

2nd person: I'd **like** to apply for a job.

1st person: **What** kind of job do you want?

2nd person: I'm an ac**coun**tant.

1st person: I'm **sure** I can help you. **Here's** an application.

2nd person: **Thank** you. **When** should I return it?

1st person: By **April** 15th.

2nd person: I'll be back on **April** 1st.

Dialog 2: IN A **SHOE** STORE

1st person: Ex**cuse** me.

2nd person *(who is not paying attention)*:   It's **my** fault. I **did**n't see you.

1st person: I **want** a pair of shoes.

2nd person: **Here's** a nice pair.

1st person: **How** much are they?

2nd person: They're **eigh**ty-five, ninety-five.

1st person: **That's** too much. **Please** show me some others.

2nd person: That's **all** we have.

1st person: I **think** I'll look around.

2nd person: **Thank** you.

Dialog 3: ACCENT MODIFICATION

1st person: **How** are you today?

2nd person: I'm **just** fine. I'd **like** to take a class.

1st person: **What's** your name?

2nd person: *(**Car**los.) My name's *(**Car**los Gomez).

1st person: **Which** class do you want?

2nd person: **Ac**cent modification.

1st person: Call **five**-five-five, two-one-one-five.

2nd person: **Thank** you. **What** time is it?

1st person: It's **ele**ven-thirty. It's **lunch** time.

2nd person: **I'll** call later.

You may insert your name here.

Dialog 4: THE **LOST** PAPER

1st person *(speaking with a fast rate):*   **Where** is that piece of paper?

2nd person: **Please** speak more slowly. I **can't** understand you.

1st person *(with a slower rate):*   **Excuse** me. I **need** to find that paper.

2nd person: **Which** paper is that?

1st person: My ad**vis**or gave me her telephone number. It's **on** that paper. I **have** to call Professor Walker.

2nd person: **What's** that paper on the floor?

1st person: **That's** the one. **Thank** you.

2nd person *(reading the paper):*   Her number is **five**-five-five, six-eight-nine-five.

1st person: **I'll** call her now.

EXERCISE 4. Adding Useful Phrases and Sentences to your *Pronunciation Notebook*

What are the phrases and sentences that you use everyday? Think of five (5) or more and add them to your *Pronunciation Notebook.* Diagram them and show them to your teacher.

SOUND ADVICE

In previous lessons, we saw how airflow and lip rounding were important for making some common American English speech sounds. We pronounced words containing sounds for which these processes are important. Now it is time to use airflow and lip rounding in sentences.

Airflow: Continuous and Interrupted

EXERCISE 5. Sentences for Practice: Continuous Airflow on the Voiceless /th/

These sentences contain a number of /th/ sounds. Remember to allow air to come through the contact that your tongue makes with your teeth. The pitch jump should occur on the word or syllable written in **boldface** type.

> I **think** I like them both.
> He was **thir**sty too.
> That's **not** a theory.
> It's the **truth**.
> **Thurs**day is my birthday.
> We **can't** think of anything.
> The **the**ater is north of Fourth Street.
> I **thought** thirteen was an unlucky number.
> The baby has **three** new teeth in her mouth.

EXERCISE 6. Sentences for Practice: Continuous Airflow on the Voiced /TH/

Continue as in Exercise 5.

> My **bro**ther and grandfather live together.
> **Ei**ther of them will do.
> They **can't** predict the weather.
> This is an**oth**er southern expression.
> They **like** those leather shoes.
> They will **meet** their father there.

EXERCISE 7. Sentences for Practice: Interrupted Airflow on /p/ and /b/

These sentences contain words with the /p/ and /b/ sounds. There are also several opportunities provided to contrast these sounds with the continuous airflow needed for /f/ and /v/.

> **Biff** planned to paint the mailbox.
> They **put** the picture above the fireplace.
> **Bea**vers build their homes in ponds.
> The **boys** brought peanuts for their friends.

We ob**served** the way Fran played the oboe.
Bev's verbal ability improved.

Lip Rounding: Slight and Tight

EXERCISE 8. Sentences for Practice: the Rounded /sh/, /zh/, /ch/, and /j/ Sounds

In these sentences, make sure that your lips are comfortably or slightly rounded (somewhat open) for these sounds.

> ***Pronunciation Note:*** Airflow for /sh/ and /zh/. These important sounds require airflow. Instead of /sh/ many speakers use /s/, and for the /zh/ they substitute /z/. When this occurs, slight lip rounding on /sh/ and /zh/ will solve the problem.

/sh/
I **wish** I could find some new shoes.
She **shopped** for a new machine.
You **should**n't go to Chicago now.
Charlotte found a shell in the ocean.

/zh/
It was a **plea**sure to visit Asia.
We **watched** the invasion on television.
The treasurer **us**ually pays the bills.
There were **ma**ny versions of the collision.

/ch/
Which teacher will cover ligatures?
Put **each** bench on the porch.
Use the remote to change the channel.
The po**ta**to chips were cheaper than the cheese.

/j/
Jonathan joined the new gym.
Jane **just** returned from Japan.
She had a **doub**le major in geology and geography.
The **judge** suggested a logical solution.

EXERCISE 9. Sentences for Practice: The Rounded /r/

The /r/ is made with about the same degree of rounding (slight) as the sounds in Exercise 8.

Robert is working for a larger firm.
Theaters offer discounts for early shows.
Runners work out every day.
The re**ports** arrived early.
The **ro**bin rested on the wire.
Jerry repairs radios in his workshop.
Our **friends** are driving to Red River.
Reindeer live in regions of the far north.
She would **ra**ther hurry than arrive late.
Where were the cars repaired?

EXERCISE 10. Sentences for Practice: The Rounded /w/

Use lip rounding that is almost closed (tight rounding) for the /w/ sound.

The **wed**ding was held on Wednesday.
Walter wondered if the money was in his wallet.
We **looked** out the window to see what the weather was like.
Where in the world is Wichita?
Where was World War I fought?
We **wan**ted to visit the wishing well.
The **wash**ing machine wasn't working very well.
What do you like about winter weather?
What language do they speak in Wales?
William was **un**aware of the news that awaited him.

LESSON 7

Asking for Information

OBJECTIVE

In this lesson, we will learn a variation of *standard intonation* for asking information questions. These questions are frequently used in interviews.

USING QUESTIONS THAT ASK FOR INFORMATION

Questions that ask for information are often called *Wh-questions* because they frequently begin with a word that starts with the letters "Wh," as in *where, what, who, which,* and *why.* The intonation pattern for these questions is like the one in Exercises 10 and 11 in Lesson 5. *Figure 7–1* helps us to see that

■ The pitch jump occurs on the Wh- word;

■ The step down must occur on every syllable that follows the pitch jump; and

■ You will use small steps down until you finally fall in pitch on the last syllable.

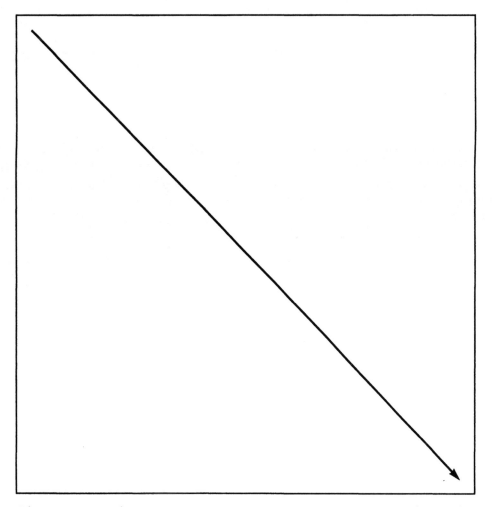

Figure 7–1. Information question intonation. Jump in pitch on the question word, then step down, and fall on the last syllable.

Example:

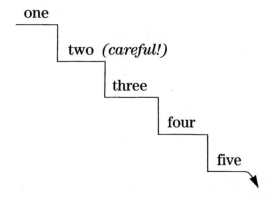

one

two *(careful!)*

three

four

five

> ***Pronunciation Note:*** Remember that in stepping down in pitch from the pitch jump, the critical step is the syllable immediately following the jump. In this example, the two is critical. If your pitch steps are too large, your pitch range will not be sufficient for the following steps, and you will not be able to fall appropriately on the last syllable.

EXERCISE 1. Diagramming Information Questions

Diagram the following sentences by showing the *jump* in pitch early in the question (on the Wh-word) and the step down to the end of the sentence, with the pitch fall on the last syllable. Do not let your pitch come up at the end of the question. Remember to place each syllable on a separate line.

1. Where do you live?

2. How much is that television set?

3. Which computer should I buy?

4. Whose turn is it to wash the dishes?

5. How long has she been working at the bookstore?

6. What happened after the accident?

7. Who went to the movies with you yesterday?

8. When does your biology class meet?

9. Why do you want to modify your accent?

10. Which street do I take to the stadium?

CONDUCTING INTERVIEWS

EXERCISE 2. The General Information Interview

Information questions may be asked to get information about another person. Ask your teacher, a friend, or another classmate for general information, using questions from the list below. When finished, you may reverse the process by answering general information questions asked by another. Write down the answers that you receive for later use in Exercise 4.

> ***Pronunciation Note:*** Because these are questions that ask for information, they must be answered with specific facts. Do not ask questions that can be answered with *yes* or *no*. We will study these kinds of questions in later lessons. They require a different pitch pattern.

General Information Questions

What's your name?

Where are you from?

What's your address?

When is your birthday?

What's your favorite _____ (color, food, book, music, class, city, vacation spot, time of the year, etc.) (You might want to ask several of these.)

How many brothers/sisters do you have?

How many countries have you visited?

What are your hobbies?

Where did you spend the summer?

What are your plans for the future?

EXERCISE 3. Focused Interviews

At times an interview may serve to obtain specific information. For example, an advisor at school may require information about education, or an employer might ask for information about work experiences. In this exercise, ask information questions from either the school *or* the job interview. Ask the same person that you interviewed in Exercise 2. Write down the answers that you receive for later use in Exercise 4.

The School Interview

What is your major?

What else are your studying in school?

How many classes are you taking?

Who are your teachers?

How long do you study every day?

When did you graduate from high school?

When will you graduate from the university?

How do you get to school?

When is your first class?

What activities do you like at school?

The Job Interview

Where do you work now?

How long have you worked there?

How many hours a day do you work?

What's your profession?

How long have you worked as a/an _____?

How much experience have you had?

Who was your last employer?

Where did you receive your training?

When were you trained?

What other jobs have you had?

EXERCISE 4. An Interview Report

Introduce the person you interviewed. Select three **general information** questions from the list in Exercise 2 and write their *answers* in the space provided. Decide where to jump in pitch and how to step down and fall at the end. Then select three questions from the **school** *or* **job** interview and write their answers. Present these as part of your interview report.

Example: This is María.

She's from **Mexico**.

Her **fa**vorite food is pizza.

She has **two** brothers and one sister.

María **loves** to read.

Her **ma**jor is botany.

She **plans** to graduate in June.

She **works** at the bookstore.

General Information

- *This is* _____. (First name of the person you interviewed; jump on the name)

- *She's/He's from* _____. (country/city/state; jump on the place)

- _____.

- _____.

- _____.

School or Job Information

- _____.

- _____.

- _____.

EXERCISE 5. Making Information Questions

Here are some answers to possible information questions. Think of an appropriate information question, one that relates to the answer, and practice proper pitch control as you jump on the Wh-word, step down on every syllable, and fall in pitch on the last syllable. As usual, jump in pitch on the syllable in **boldface** type.

Example: Last **Thurs**day.   <u>When did they leave on their vacation?</u>

1. To**mor**row. _____

2. **Tok**yo. _____

3. My **grand**father. _____

4. **Thir**ty-nine (39) cents. _____

5. Chi**ca**go. _____

6. Bi**ol**ogy. _____

7. **Af**ter class. _____

8. The **doc**tor. _____

9. $99.95 (**Nine**ty-nine, ninety-five). _____

10. **Swim**ming. _____

11. **Mine**. _____

12. Ko**re**a. _____

13. The **tea**cher's. _____

14. 12 (**twelve**). _____

15. Because he's **sick**. _____

16. Your **pass**port. _____

17. **Piz**za. _____

18. At 6 (**six**) o'clock. _____

19. **Five**-thousand dollars. _____

20. **Fif**ty. _____

EXERCISE 6. Diagramming

Select any *five* of the above and diagram the information questions (not their answers) using the correct pattern.

1.

2.

3.

4.

5.

SOUND ADVICE

Airflow and Lip Rounding

In previous lessons, we studied continuous and interrupted airflow. We also learned about slight and tight lip rounding. These processes were practiced in both words and sentences. In this lesson, we will use these important processes in the context of dialogs that contain words with sounds that use airflow and lip rounding.

DIALOG 1: THANKS A LOT!

Person 1: I've been **thin**king about the Thanksgiving vacation.

Person 2: **Why** are you thinking about a vacation? This is the **first** week of school.

Person 1: That's e**xac**tly why I'm thinking about a vacation. I **thought** I'd do something fun.

Person 2: **Where** do you think you'll go?

Person 1: I **thought** I'd go to Athens. **Think** about going with me. **You** could pay the bills.

Person 2: That's what **you** think. I have **o**ther plans.

Person 1: Then I'll **go** without you. **Thanks** a lot!

Dialog 2: WHERE'S THE LIBRARY?

Person 1: **Par**don me. **Where's** the library? I've been **sear**ching for hours.

Person 2: **I'm** sorry. I **did**n't hear you.

Person 1: I'm **try**ing to remember where the library is. I **have**n't been here for years. I **thought** the library was right around here.

Person 2: You're **very** close. But you **can't** see it from here.

Person 1: There are **too** many trees.

Person 2: The **lib**rary is around the corner. It's **near** that red brick building. **Walk** over there.

Person 1: Per**haps** I should drive my car. **Now** I can borrow the books I need for my work.

Person 2: I should **warn** you. There is **no**where to park in that area.

Dialog 3: THE TOOTH FAIRY

Person 1: My **bro**ther has some loose teeth. **What** do you know about the Tooth Fairy?

Person 2: There is a **fun**ny theory about children's teeth.

Person 1: **What's** the theory? I **need** to know something about it.

Person 2: The **child** puts her teeth under her pillow. The **Tooth** Fairy comes and takes the teeth. The child receives **mo**ney for the teeth.

Person 1: **How** much are they worth?

Person 2: **That** depends on how many teeth there are.

Person 1: There are **three** of them.

Person 2: They are worth at least **thir**ty cents each.

Person 1: My **grand**father has false teeth. **How** much are those teeth worth?

Person 2: You're **lucky**! False teeth aren't worth **any**thing to the Tooth Fairy.

Dialog 4: THE MARATHON

Person 1: I **might** run in a marathon this year.

Person 2: **How** far do you run in a marathon?

Person 1: Somewhere between **twen**ty and thirty miles.

Person 2: That's **rea**lly a rugged run.

Person 1: **Right.** I'm **sure** I'm ready for a long race.

Person 2: **Why** run that far?

Person 1: I've been **wor**king out every day. I run **rough**ly thirteen miles.

Person 2: That **does**n't sound far enough for a marathon.

Person 1: That's **half** a marathon. I'll run the **se**cond half of a marathon.

Person 2: It **does**n't work like that. You'd **bet**ter keep running.

EXERCISE 7. Review

Circle the correct answer from the *italicized* words in the following statements.

1. When someone says *tink* for *think*, the problem is primarily *lip rounding / airflow*.

2. The sounds /h/, /s/, and /f/ require *lip rounding / airflow*.

3. The sounds /sh/, /zh/, /ch/, and /j/ are made with *relaxed lips / rounded lips*.

4. The lips should be *rounded / not rounded* for the /l/ sound.

5. The /r/ sound in American English requires the bottom lip to be *rounded / not rounded*.

6. The lips should be rounded for /w/ / /v/.

7. The lips should be *rounded / not rounded* for /ch/.

8. The /sh/ sound is made with airflow and *lip rounding / no lip rounding*.

9. The /r/ sound is made with *slight / tight* lip rounding.

10. The /w/ sound is made with *slight / tight* lip rounding.

LESSON 8

Determining Where to Jump in Pitch

OBJECTIVE

In this lesson you will learn what kinds of words in American English sentences have a high or low probability for the pitch jump for standard intonation. You will also review –s endings on plural, possessive, and present tense words.

STANDARD INTONATION

Standard intonation refers to the *walk, jump, step, fall* pattern that is most frequently used by speakers of American English. It is the pattern that will always "work" in the language. As you study this lesson, keep these points in mind concerning standard intonation:

- Jump in pitch on a meaningful word in the sentence.

- Jump in pitch on the prominent syllable of the word selected for the pitch jump.

- The word selected for the pitch jump will usually occur early in the sentence.

- Jump only one time in short sentences.

- Jump on the word containing the *new* information in the sentence.

WORDS WITH A HIGH PROBABILITY OF RECEIVING THE PITCH JUMP

Certain kinds of words in American English have a higher probability of receiving the pitch jump than other words. These are called *content* words because they are important to the meaning of what we say.

Information-Asking Question Words (See Lesson 7)

Some examples are: *who* (name), *what* (thing), *where* (place), *when* (time), *why* (reason), *how* (manner), *whose* (person's), *which* (thing), *how much* (quantity), and *how long* (time or distance).

EXERCISE 1. Question Words

Practice these questions that ask for information. Jump in pitch on the word or syllable in **boldface** type.

Who are the authors of this book?
Why did the car run out of gas?
Where are they going to shop?
What do you want for dinner?
How much does it cost?
When does baseball season begin?

Negative Words

Some examples are *no, not, can't, won't, none,* and *never.*

 EXERCISE 2. Words with Negative Meaning

Practice these sentences. Jump in pitch on the negative word.

We **can't** do our homework. (Compare: **We** can do our homework.)
Mary **does**n't like spinach.
They **are**n't going to the picnic.
I'm **not** finished.
None of the children wanted ice cream.
We **ne**ver have enough time.

> *Pronunciation Note:* Do not increase loudness on negative words unless you want to make them very definite, as in *I said I'm NOT going!*

Words of Manner and Time (known as adverbs)

Manner: *quickly, carefully, very, slowly*

Time: *just, while, always, seldom*

 EXERCISE 3. Adverbs

Practice these sentences that contain words of manner and time.

We **just** finished studying.
John **al**ways does his work.
She **slow**ly walked to the exit.
I **real**ly want to sing in the choir.
She was **very** happy to see us.

Words for Persons, Places, and Things (known as subject nouns and subject pronouns)

Persons: *John, Mary, fire fighter*

Places: *New York, Baltimore, Kansas*

Things: *book, car, engineering*

Pronouns (substitute words for nouns): *I, you, he, she, we, they*

EXERCISE 4. Nouns

Practice these sentences jumping in pitch on the word or syllable in **boldface** type.

Fred is writing her a letter.
He is waiting for a bus.
Mary and Alice want pie for dessert.
The **car** was damaged.
A **nic**kel is worth five pennies.
Paris is my favorite city. (Pronounce *fav'rite* with two syllables.)

Action Words (known as main verbs)

Examples: *run, walk, sing, speak, jump, fall*

EXERCISE 5. Verbs

Practice these sentences that have the pitch jump on the main verb.

She **ran** to the garage.
They **played** in the park.
Speak so that people can understand you.
Read for relaxation.
Jump on important words.
He **fought** for justice.

Words that "Point" (known as demonstratives)

Examples: *this, that, these, those*

Exercise 6. Demonstrative Words

Practice these sentences that emphasize how the pitch jump occurs on words that "point."

That one belongs to my neighbor.
I have **this** one.
Those (books) are mine. (Words in parentheses may be omitted)

These (insects) bother me.
They want to study **this** lesson.
These are big enough.

Words that Describe (known as adjectives)

Examples: *red, blue, three, large, small*

EXERCISE 7. Adjectives

Practice these sentences in which the pitch jump occurs on words that describe.

The **red** car belongs to John.
There are **three** books on the desk.
The **small** tree is a maple.
It's a **big** city.
She gave a **won**derful report.
It's a **great** day for a picnic.

WORDS WITH A LOW PROBABILITY OF RECEIVING THE PITCH JUMP

Some words, called *structure* words because they are important to the grammar of American English, do <u>not</u> ordinarily receive the jump in pitch. Here are some examples.

Articles: *a/an, the*

> *Pronunciation Note:* The article *a* occurs before words that begin with consonant sounds; *an* occurs before words that begin with vowel sounds. The article *the* also has two pronunciations. Before consonant sounds, the article is pronounced with the neutral vowel, /ə/. When *the* occurs before words that begin with a vowel sound, it is pronounced with /ee/.
>
> Compare: *a book, a car, a visit*
>
> To: *an apple, an architect, an eagle*; and
>
> Compare: *the book, the car, the visit*
>
> To: *the apple, the architect, the eagle*

EXERCISE 8. Articles

Practice these sentences, jumping in pitch on the word or syllable in **boldface** type. Do not jump on articles (underlined).

The **boy** had an apple.
That's a **real**ly cute puppy.
I have a **pen**cil and an eraser.
The **book** you wanted is here.
The **ar**chitect designed it.
The **ea**gle is a bird.

Words that Connect (known as conjunctions)

Examples: *and, or, but*

EXERCISE 9. Conjunctions

Practice these sentences jumping in pitch on the word or syllable in **boldface** type. Do not jump on the underlined conjunction.

Mary and Bill are my friends.
She wants **cof**fee or tea.
Sam has **nine** dollars but needs twelve.
They were **tired** so they left.
I went **home** and read a book.
He **hur**ried but he was late.

"Helping" Verbs (or support verbs, verbs that are used with other, more important verbs)

Examples: *can, may, will, should, is, are, was, were*

EXERCISE 10. Helping Verbs

Practice jumping in pitch on the word in **boldface** type, not on the underlined helping verb.

Ann can play the flute.
You'll **like** this class. (*will* may be contracted as *'ll*)

He's **run**ning for president. (*is* may be contracted as *'s*)
He did **not** want it. (compare: He **did**n't want it.)
Students should study every day.

Other Pronouns (not pronouns that can serve as the subject of the sentence)

Examples: *me, you, him, her, it, us, them*

EXERCISE 11. Other Pronouns

Practice these sentences. Do not jump on the underlined pronoun.

The **ban**ker gave me a loan.
Wendy went with us.
Sally wanted them to call her.
Their **pit**cher threw him the ball.
When will it be ready?
Who will go with us?

Prepositions (words that connect nouns in time or space)

Examples: *in, on, under, around, over*

EXERCISE 12. Prepositions

In practicing these sentences, do not jump on the underlined preposition.

The **stamps** are in the drawer.
We **drove** around the block.
The **air**plane flew over the city.
The **car** on the left is mine.
Look under the table.
How far is it to the market?

> ***Pronunciation Note:*** When prepositions function as adverbs, they may receive the pitch jump, for example, *it's **on** the floor.*

DIALOGS FOR PRACTICE

Dialogs provide a valuable learning experience for us because they are both conversational and practical. Notice that the pitch jumps occur early and on important words. You will also notice that in some sentences, the pitch jump will occur on *new information* introduced into the conversation by one of the speakers. Words containing new information are frequently used for the pitch jump. In Dialog 1, *nearly*, *game*, and *lost* are excellent examples of new information.

In the first of these two dialogs, jump in pitch on the word or syllable in each sentence in **boldface** type. These are high probability words for the pitch jump because they carry the meaning of the sentence or introduce new information into the conversation. Practice the sentences until you can control the *walk, jump, step, fall* pattern expressed in each. In the second dialog, select the most probable word in each sentence and underline it. Then walk to that word and jump in pitch on it. Don't forget to step down on each syllable that follows, and fall at the end of the sentence. Be prepared to present these dialogs.

DIALOG 1: **DON'T** BE LATE!

Person 1:   **When** will you be ready?

Person 2:   I'm **near**ly ready to go.

Person 1:   I **real**ly don't want to be late.

Person 2:   You're **never** late. You **just** like to worry.

Person 1:   The **game** starts at 7:30. I'd **like** to be there by 7 o'clock.

Person 2.   **OK. Let's** go. **What's** the matter now?

Person 1:   I've **lost** the tickets.

DIALOG 2: AN IM**POR**TANT VISITOR.

Person 1:   That must have been an important call. You seem really nervous.

Person 2:   We need to get this place cleaned up. I'll wash the dishes. You sweep the floor.

Person 1:   I want to watch T.V. I'll help you in an hour.

Person 2:   You'd better help me now. We're in big trouble.

Person 1:   Who was on the phone?

Person 2:   Your mother!

Person 1:   Why didn't you say so? Get busy!

SHOW AND TELL

We often have to talk about things or demonstrate how something works. This activity will provide you with a strategy for doing this. We all have a favorite object that we like to talk about. For this activity

- Find something interesting, such as a souvenir from a trip, something you collect, a picture, or something characteristic of your culture.
- Write a description, about 10 sentences in length.
- Keep the sentences short for better control.
- Mark where you will jump in pitch.
- Show your marked sentences to your teacher.
- Practice your approved report until you can control each sentence.
- Try to memorize your *show and tell*.
- Remember: *walk, jump, step, fall*.
- Prepare to answer information-asking questions about your report.
- Present your *show and tell*.

EXERCISE 13. Review

Answer the following questions.

1. In American English, standard intonation is a pitch pattern based on

   _____, _____ , _____, and _____.

2. Jump in pitch on a (circle) *meaningful / meaningless* word in the sentence.

3. Jump in pitch on the (circle) *weak / prominent* syllable of the word selected for the pitch jump.

4. Jump in pitch on the (circle) *old / new* information in the sentence.

5. Decide whether these words have a high or a low probability of having the pitch jump. Write *high* or *low* in the space provided.

    a. When . . .?   _____

    b. and   _____

    c. can   _____

    d. they   _____

    e. not   _____

    f. a   _____

    g. is   _____

    h. them   _____

    i. just   _____

    j. Bill   _____

    k. always   _____

    l. the   _____

SOUND ADVICE

The Pronunciation of –s Word Endings

American English has a relatively uncomplicated grammar. There are few word endings. However, when word endings are used, they should be pronounced. You have probably heard that "–s word endings" are used to

- Form plurals out of singular nouns (*book* becomes *books*)
- Make nouns possessive (*John* becomes *John's*)
- Make verbs correspond to a singular subject in present time *(He runs)*

You also have probably heard that

- If the last consonant in the word is voiceless you add a pronounced /s/
- If the last consonant in the word is voiced, you add a pronounced /z/

■ If the last consonant in the word is /s, z, sh, ch, or j/, add the reduced vowel /ə/, plus /z/, as in *dresses, raises, dishes, churches,* and *judges.*

> ***Pronunciation Note:*** Many speakers of American English do not apply these rules strictly. They will tend to pronounce final /z/ as /s/, so that words like *price* and *prize* sound very similar except for the length of the vowel (it is longer in *prize,* as explained in Lesson 13).

In this lesson, we will practice adding a final syllable ("–es") on words that end in /s, z, sh, ch, and j/. Speakers of American English as another language will usually require additional practice with this aspect of –s word endings.

EXERCISE 14. Plural Nouns

Practice these nouns that require an added syllable.

dish (əz)	toothbrush (əz)
rose	license
peach	hose
prize	badge
page	cage
bus	bench
watch	class

EXERCISE 15. Plural Noun Practice

Make these nouns plural by adding /əz/ (neutral vowel plus /z/ or /s/). Use the following dialog. The teacher will select a word from the list and pronounce it without the ending. The student uses the plural ending. Jump in pitch on the word or syllable written in **boldface** type.

Teacher: *dish*

Student 1:   **How** many dish+/əz/ do we need?

Student 2:   **Three** dish+/əz/. We need **three** dish+/əz/.

Student 1:   I **on**ly have two dish+/əz/.

Student 2:   We **need** to get more dish+/əz/.

(Student 1 then selects another word from the list.)

EXERCISE 16. Possessive Nouns

Practice these nouns with the added syllable.

George (əz)	Wes (əz)
Madge	Joyce
Elvis	Liz
Louise	Santa Claus
the judge	Trish
the coach	Mitch
Josh	the witch
Marsh	Tish

EXERCISE 17. Possessive Noun Practice

Make these nouns possessive by adding /əz/ (neutral vowel plus /z/). In using this dialog, select one of the persons listed in Exercise 16. Then select one of the options (what the person owns).

Options: coat sweater glove watch hat

Student 1: **Whose** coat *(one of the options)* is this?

Student 2: **George**+/əz/. *(a person selected from the list in Exercise 16)* It's **George**+/əz/ coat.

Student 1: **Where** should I put George+/əz/ coat?

(Student 2 continues with another selection from the options.)

EXERCISE 18. Present Time Verbs

Practice the words in this list. They require the addition of the neutral vowel with /z/ (or /s/).

teach (əz)	watch (əz)
advise	wash
fish	publish
coach	manage
discuss	exercise

EXERCISE 19. Present Time Verb Practice

Change these verbs into present tense singular verbs. Add /əz/ (neutral vowel plus /z/ or /s/). Use this dialog. The teacher selects a word from the list and pronounces it without the ending. The student uses the plural ending. Jump in pitch on the word or syllable written in **boldface** type.

Teacher: *teach*

Student 1:   **Mary** teach+/əz/.

Student 2:   **Teach**+/əz/. **Who** teach+/əz/?

Student 1:   **Mary** teach+/əz/. She teach+/əz/ on **Tues**day.

Student 2:   John **al**so teach+/əz/ on Tuesday.

(Student 1 then selects another word from the list in Exercise 18.)

LESSON 9

"The Fox and the Grapes": A Passage for Practice

OBJECTIVE

In this lesson you will practice a strategy for telling a story. First, you will determine where the pitch jumps occur. Then you will practice the problem words used in the story. (In the next lesson we will complete our analysis and practice of this famous story.) We will also review the pronunciation of past tense verbs.

THE STORY OF "THE FOX AND THE GRAPES"

EXERCISE 1. Determining Pitch Jumps in a Fable Written by Aesop

With the help of your teacher, decide where the pitch jumps occur in this story and underline all the words or syllables.

Mister Fox was just about famished. He was thirsty, too. So he crept into a vineyard. The sun-ripened grapes were hanging on a trellis above the ground. They were too high for him to reach. He ran and jumped for the nearest bunch of grapes. But he missed. Again and again he tried. Still he could not reach the luscious prize. Soon he became very tired. Worn out by his efforts, he left the vineyard. "Well," he muttered, "I never really wanted those grapes anyway. I'm sure they are sour. They probably have worms in them, too!"

The moral of the story is: We might not like what we cannot easily attain.

EXERCISE 2. Diagramming

Now that you have determined where to jump in pitch, diagram each sentence from this story in *walk, jump, step, fall* (standard) intonation. Then practice each sentence until it sounds natural.

Mister Fox was just about famished.

He was thirsty, too.

So he crept into a vineyard.

The sun-ripened grapes were hanging on a trellis above the ground.

They were too high for him to reach.

He ran and jumped for the nearest bunch of grapes.

But he missed.

Again and again he tried.

Still he could not reach the luscious prize.

Soon he became very tired.

Worn out by his efforts, he left the vineyard.

"Well," he muttered, "I never really wanted those grapes anyway.

I'm sure they are sour.

They probably have worms in them, too!"

The moral of the story is: We might not like what we cannot easily attain.

EXERCISE 3. Learning to Pronounce the Problem Words in "The Fox and The Grapes."

a. Difficult Words. Here are some of the words that students find difficult to pronounce. Practice each word, jumping in pitch on the important (stressed) syllable. Check a dictionary if you are not sure where the pitch jump is.

thirsty	vineyard	grapes	sour
nearest	muttered	trellis	worms
bunch	anyway	those	easily
famished	probably	luscious	worn
Mister	sun-ripened	crept	again

Fox	tired	very	wanted
jumped	hanging	sure	efforts
ground	reach	still	missed

b. **Practicing Difficult Words.** Use each problem word in these phrases. You may treat these sentences as a dialog for additional practice.

Person 1: **How** do you say the word _____? (Jump on *How*)

Person 2: _____. You say _____. (Jump on the "word")

Person 1: _____. I **like** the word _____. (Jump on *like*)

Person 2: The **word** _____ could be useful. (Jump on *word*)

c. **Practicing the Story**. Now practice the story, attending to your pronunciation of these words *and* to the pitch pattern of each sentence.

> ***Pronunciation Note 1:*** The "tt" in *muttered* is pronounced as /d/. A /t/ between vowels is frequently pronounced as a /d/.
>
> ***Pronunciation Note 2:*** When /t/ occurs after /n/, as in *wanted*, and the syllable containing /t/ does not contain the pitch jump, the /t/ may not be pronounced in American English. Examples: *enter, center, county, dental, printer, advantage, Atlantic, romantic, Santa Claus, interview, interval, parental, accidental, horizontal, governmental, documentary, oriental, winter.* But the /t/ is pronounced in: *integrity, contempt, continue, container, contestant, contemporary.* In these words, the pitch jump occurs in the syllable with /t/.

SOUND ADVICE

The Pronunciation of Past Tense Endings

In American English "–ed" is added to regular verbs for past tense. This ending may be pronounced in three ways: as a /t/, /d/, or as an additional syllable, pronounced with the neutral vowel /ə/ plus /d/. Remember that the /t/ is voiceless and the /d/ is voiced. If the sound preceding the past tense ending is voiceless, the /t/ is used. Therefore, *cooked* ends with a /t/ sound because /k/ is voiceless. In *rubbed* a /d/ is used because /b/ is voiced. If the verb already ends with a "d" or a "t," as in *need* or *want*, we add another syllable— "–ed," as in *needed* and *wanted*. These rules always apply when a regular past tense verb is said alone or at the end of a sentence. Many verbs are irregular and do not fit this logical pattern, however.

EXERCISE 4. Regular Verbs for Past Tense Practice

a. Practice with Past Tense Endings. The pronunciation of the past tense ending, usually written "–ed," is shown above the top three columns of words in this exercise. Practice saying each word with and without the past tense ending. In words of two syllables, jump on the syllable written in **boldface** type. Remember that adding an extra syllable does not change where you jump in pitch.

/d/	/t/	/əd/
close	slice	count
fill	type	mend
mail	kick	need
serve	an**nounce**	grade
glue	**fi**nish	rate
move	tape	want
scrub	push	add
en**joy**	bake	skate

b. Deciding How to Pronounce Past Tense Endings. In the following two columns, decide which form of the past tense ending is required for each word and write it in the space provided. Practice saying each word.

?		?	
jump	____	dis**cuss**	____
wait	____	**o**pen	____
mutter	____	raid	____
need	____	play	____
work	____	wrap	____
de**cide**	____	try	____
miss	____	pat	____
create	____	use	____
re**spond**	____	re**pair**	____

EXERCISE 5. A Practice Dialog

Using the words in Exercise 4, the teacher will say the word *without* the past tense ending. The student will add the appropriate past tense ending: /t/, /d/, or /–əd/, and use the word in the dialog. The teacher will select a verb from the list of regular verbs.

      Example: Teacher: **Slice.**

Student 1:   **How** do you say the word *sliced?*

Student 2:   **Sliced.** You say **sliced.**

Student 1:   **Sliced.** I **like** the word *sliced.*

Student 2:   The **word** *sliced* could be useful.

(Student 1 then selects another verb from the list in Exercise 4a.)

EXERCISE 6. Longer Regular Past Time Verbs for Practice

In this exercise, decide if the verb requires /t/, /d/, or /əd/. Then write the appropriate ending in the space provided. Practice saying each word. As usual, the syllable receiving the pitch jump is written in **boldface** type.

      Examples: initiate   _əd_ **pur**chase   _t_

> ***Pronunciation Note:*** Notice that some of these verbs end with a "silent e." In these cases, the consonant before the "e" determines which past time ending will be used. Notice that the word *speculate* ends with a "silent e." Therefore, the "t" will determine that /əd/ should be used to produce *speculated.*

re**mem**ber	_____	pre**reg**ister	_____
ex**pect**	_____	**for**mat	_____
celebrate	_____	pro**nounce**	_____
con**sult**	_____	reim**burse**	_____

compre**hend** ____   de**ve**lop ____

com**man**d ____   dis**co**ver ____

credit ____   ac**com**plish ____

con**gra**tulate ____   **re**cognize ____

pro**vi**de ____   con**ti**nue ____

LESSON 10

Using Ligatures and Blends

OBJECTIVE

In this lesson you will learn to use *ligatures* and *blends*. Ligatures are formed when a consonant at the end of a word moves to form a syllable with a following vowel that begins the next word. A blend is formed when two vowels or two consonants are joined in speech.

Remember These Things as You Work on Ligatures and Blends:

- We do not speak in individuals sounds, as in *c-a-t*.

- We speak in sounds combined into syllables, as in *cat*.

- Use *walk, jump, step, fall* intonation.

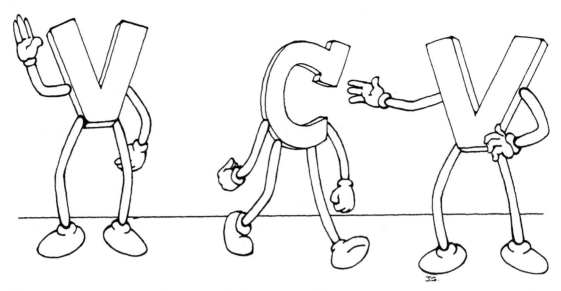

Figure 10–1. Making ligatures. When a word begins with a vowel the preceding consonant will move to it.

MAKING LIGATURES

Pay attention to the ends of words in American English. They are very important and are usually pronounced. The ends of words carry more grammatical information than the beginning of words in American English, as we have seen in Lessons 8 and 9 in this text. If you do not pronounce the ends of words or do not use ligatures and blends, speech may become difficult to understand because important information is left out.

Because we speak in syllables, each syllable will usually contain a consonant followed by a vowel. Therefore, for speech, the general pattern is Consonant-Vowel, Consonant-Vowel, Consonant-Vowel, and so on. If a syllable in a word ends with a consonant, and if the next word begins with a vowel, the consonant will usually move to the vowel that follows (Avery & Ehrlich, 1992; Temperley, 1987). These "links" are called *ligatures*. See *Figure 10–1*.

Examples: thanks a lot = **thank**-sa-lot
We clean it = we-**clea**-nit
We cleaned it = we-**clean**-dit

EXERCISE 1. Phrases and Sentences with Ligatures

Circle the ligatures. Then practice these phrases and sentences. Jump on the syllable or word written in **boldface** type.

Example: Sam opened it.

ten o'clock	That's **all**.	**Here** it is.	**Turn** it off.
after awhile	It's **easy**.	**Look** at it.	**Give** it up.
his **uncle**	**again** and again	**looked** at it	**John** is angry.

> ***Pronunciation Note:*** Remember that a /t/ between vowels is commonly pronounced as /d/, as in the words *letter* and *better*. In making ligatures, a /t/ may also occur between vowels even when they are in different words. In the sentence, ***Here*** *it is*, the /t/ is actually between the vowel /i/ of *it* and /i/ of *is*, and is pronounced ***He**-ri-dis*. (The final letter of *here* is not pronounced.)

EXERCISE 2. Finding Ligatures

Circle all of the ligatures in these sentences. Then practice saying each sentence (a) with appropriate intonation by jumping on the syllable or word in **boldface** type, and (b) with the ligatures joined in a syllable. The number at the end of each sentence tells you how many ligatures to expect.

Example: Brad opened a jar of applesauce. (4)

1. His **o**ther suit is in the closet. (3)

2. **Don't** come for us until I call you. (3)

3. **Sam** is going to meet us this afternoon. (3)

4. The **news** is on at eleven o'clock. (5)

5. **Let's** have a party with all of our friends. (4)

6. **When** are Agnes and you leaving for Alaska? (4)

7. **How** much is it when you call India? (3)

8. He has an ap**point**ment this afternoon. (3)

9. **I'd** like a dish of ice cream. (3)

10. They put **a**pples and oranges in every box. (5)

MAKING BLENDS

Vowel Blends

Ligatures are formed by a consonant and a vowel. Blends are formed when two vowels occur together in speech, Consonant-Vowel + Vowel-Consonant. It is relatively easy to learn to join a consonant and a following vowel into one syllable. However, blending two vowels together is much more difficult (see *Figure 10–2*). Here are the rules:

■ If the first vowel is rounded (/uw, u, o/ and /aw/), a /w/-sound is spoken before the following vowel:

Sue is . . . becomes **Sue** (w)-is . . .
No apples . . . **No** (w)-apples
How old . . . **How** (w)-old

■ For all other vowels (unrounded), a /y/-sound is added to the following vowel:

He is . . . becomes **He** (y)-is . . .
I am . . . becomes **I** (y)-am . . .
the apple . . . becomes the (**y**)-**a**pple
fly around . . . becomes **fly** (y)-around

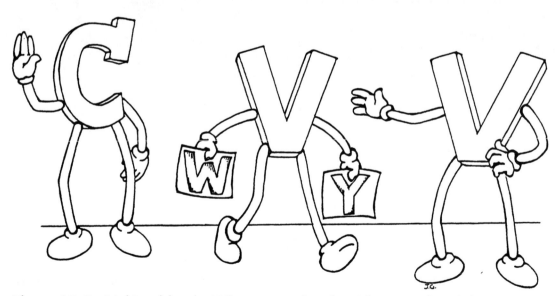

Figure 10–2. Making blends. When a word ends with a vowel and the next one begins with a vowel, either /y/ or /w/ will serve to blend them together.

EXERCISE 3. Finding Vowel Blends

Circle all the vowel blends in these phrases. Then write in a "w" or a "y" as required by the blend. As usual, jump in pitch on the syllable or word in **boldface** type.

> ***Pronunciation Note:*** Sometimes the spelling of words may help us to know whether to use a /w/ or a /y/ sound. The word *how* in *how old* tells us that the vowel of *how* is rounded. Therefore the word *old* will begin with the /w/ sound. Other examples are:
>
> **row** over
>
> **cow** is
>
> **blow** in
>
> Likewise, there are words that end with the letter /y/ that tell us we should pronounce the following vowel with this sound so that *fly around* becomes *fly (y)-around*. Some other examples are:
>
> **they** are (the "y" blends to the word *are*)
>
> **say** it
>
> **sky** is
>
> **boy** is

Example: Su**e** answered.

We are.	**I** am.	**yel**low apples
Do it.	so **I**	**throw** out
Who is?	we **all**	**shoe** is
She is.	you **add**	**know** about

Exercise 4. Finding Blends in Sentences

Circle all the vowel blends in these sentences, then write in the "w" or "y" as required by the blend. The number of blends follows each sentence. You will also want to circle the ligatures in these sentences in a different color.

Example: We are too early. (2)

(above "are" is "y", above "too" is "w")

1. **Sue** is going with us? (1)

2. **Who** answered the other phone? (2)

3. They **aren't** too angry. (2)

4. She **only** wants to eat yellow apples. (3)

5. The artist **always** wants to arrange her work. (2)

6. I **hope** she will be on time. (1)

7. We **each** need a book of our own. (1)

8. I **hope** the agency accepts my offer. (3)

9. **I'll** be over after I eat dinner. (2)

10. They **always** see every airplane in the airport. (4)

Consonant Blends

If the same consonant sounds (or very similar sounds) occur next to each other, they will blend together to form a single sound. In *I'll call later*, the /l/ in *call* is followed by the /l/ of *later*. These blend to form one /l/ sound, as in *I'll ca-later*. Some other examples are:

His-zip code

next-to

red-door

with-them

EXERCISE 5. Finding Consonant Blends

Circle all the consonant blends in these phrases. Then practice them, jumping in pitch on the syllables or words in **boldface** type.

Example: more radios

never really   **let** Tim

big goat   **bad** dog

walk carefully   some **more**

hot tea   **stop** pushing.

EXERCISE 6. Finding Consonant Blends in Sentences

Circle all the consonant blends in these sentences. Then pronounce them in the usual manner. There are also other ligatures and blends in these sentences. Can you locate them?

> **Example:** Janette took care of Victor.

1. **I** need some more. (1)

2. The **big** game is this Saturday. (2)

3. They had **done** their report. (2)

4. **Jack** came home at ten o'clock. (2)

5. They **ne**ver really understood. (1)

6. We had **dra**ma last term. (2)

LIGATURES AND BLENDS AND THE H- PRONOUNS:
HE, HIM, HIS, HER, HERS, HERSELF, HIMSELF

There are several pronouns that begin with /h/ such as *he, her, himself,* and *herself.* These pronouns usually follow another word in a sentence and may not be pronounced with the beginning /h/ sound. When this happens, these rules apply.

■ For these /h/ pronouns, the "h" is often replaced by the consonant from the word before to form a ligature.

Thank him *becomes* **Than**-kim

Thank her *becomes* **Than**-ker

John has his *becomes* **John**-ha-sis (ziz)

She made it herself *becomes* **She**-ma-di-der-self

Took her *becomes* **Too**-ker

Soon he left *becomes* **Soo**-ne-left

If he *becomes* **I**-fe

■ If the word before the omitted "h" ends with a rounded vowel, then a blend will occur with /w/:

Give it to her *becomes* **Gi**-vi-to-wer

Show it to him *becomes* **Sho**-wi-to-wim

To his *becomes* To-**wis** (wiz)

Show her *becomes* **Sho**-wer

So he left *becomes* So-we-**left**

■ If the word before the omitted "h" ends with an unrounded vowel, then a blend with the /y/-sound will occur:

See him *becomes* **See**-yim

See her *becomes* **See**-yer

by himself *becomes* b(y)-yim**self**

be herself *becomes* be-yer-**self**

> ***Pronunciation Note:*** Ligatures and blends are made very smoothly and softly. They are not pronounced very precisely. Continued practice will soon result in making them sound natural.

EXERCISE 7. Working with H- Pronouns

Draw a line through the /h/ to show that it is not pronounced. Then circle all the ligatures and blends that result. For the blends, write in the "w" (rounded vowel) or "y" (unrounded vowel) that occurs. Practice the sentences. Remember to jump in pitch on the word or syllable in **boldface** type.

Example: John **gave** her a ride to her house.

1. I've **seen** her new car.

2. They **made** him go with her.

3. **Bob** went back to his room.

4. **Joan** let him buy her lunch.

5. **Bill** wanted her to be his tutor.

6. **Ken** helped her do her homework.

7. They **said** he would do it himself.

8. **Sue** sent the box to herself.

> ***Pronunciation Note:*** In sentence 4, we pronounce the /t/ in *let* as a /d/ because it is between vowels when the /h/ is lost.

MARKING PITCH JUMPS, LIGATURES, AND BLENDS

EXERCISE 8. Putting It All Together

a. Pitch Jumps. Using the information on high probability words for the pitch jump from Lesson 8, <u>underline</u> an appropriate word (or syllable within an important word) in these sentences and practice the intonation pattern. When in doubt, jump on the earliest important word in the sentence.

Example: I <u>don't</u> like it when the opera is sad.

1. He asked us a few other questions.

2. Sally is driving her car to Arizona.

3. Who left the keys on the desk?

4. He wants no part in our plan.

5. Sue read novels in her English class.

6. Pam and her sister took the same anatomy class.

7. How old is the administration building?

8. I am anxious to be on her thesis committee.

9. How far is it to our apartment?

10. I wanted to thank him for all he did on Monday.

b. **Ligatures.** Now circle all the <u>ligatures</u> in these ten sentences. Don't forget the "h" pronouns.

   Example: I don't li(ke it) when the opera is sad.

c. **Blends.** Now circle all the vowel and consonant blends and add "w" or "y" as appropriate.

   Example: I don't like it when th(eyo)per(ayi)(s s)ad.

EXERCISE 9. A Dialog for Practice

For additional practice, turn to Lesson 8 and the dialog titled, "An Important Visitor." Circle all ligatures and blends, marking the blends with "w" or "y" as necessary.

EXERCISE 10. Marking Ligatures and Blends in the Story of "The Fox and the Grapes"

Mark all of the pitch jumps from memory. Then find and circle all of the ligatures. Next, locate the blends. Write in the /w/ or /y/ sound as appropriate for the blends.

"THE FOX AND THE GRAPES"

Marking Jumps, Ligatures, and Blends

Mister Fox was just about famished. He was thirsty, too. So he crept into a vineyard. The sun-ripened grapes were hanging on a trellis above the ground. They were too high for him to reach. He ran and jumped for the nearest bunch of grapes. But he missed. Again and again he tried. Still he could not reach the luscious prize. Soon he became very tired. Worn out by his efforts, he left the vineyard. "Well," he muttered, "I never really wanted those grapes anyway. I'm sure they are sour.

They probably have worms in them, too!"

The moral of the story is: We might not like what we cannot easily attain.

EXERCISE 11. Review

Circle the correct answer (one of the *italicized* words) in these statements.

1. A *ligature / blend* is formed when a consonant sound that ends a word moves to the vowel sound that begins the next word.

2. A *ligature / blend* is formed when a vowel sound ends a word and a vowel sound begins the next word.

3. When a word ends with a rounded vowel, the blend to the vowel sound beginning the next word is made with a *w sound / y sound*.

4. Ligatures and blends may also occur with *nouns / pronouns* that begin with the letter "h."

5. For "h" pronouns in ligatures and blends, the "h" is *pronounced / not pronounced*.

6. If a word ends with a vowel sound which is not rounded, the blend to the vowel sound beginning the next word is made with a *w sound / y sound*.

SOUND ADVICE

The Pronunciation of Word Endings

EXERCISE 12. Regular Past Tense Verbs: Sentences for Practice

In Lesson 9, we studied past tense verbs. Now we will practice verbs in sentences. As usual, jump on the word written in **boldface** type. Also, remember to mark and use ligatures and blends.

1. The **chil**dren packed their bags for camp.

2. We **washed** the dishes carefully.

3. **Last** summer they climbed the mountain.

4. The **plane** landed at the airport on time.

5. I **cleaned** the house last week.

6. **Jim** taped his photograph to the wall.

7. The secretary typed **ten** letters before going to lunch.

8. **E**veryone in the family smiled for the portrait.

9. We **ska**ted at the roller skating rink yesterday.

10. She served **ice** cream and cake for dessert.

EXERCISE 13. Word Endings with –s: Sentences for Practice

In Lesson 8, we studied the various uses of –s endings in American English. Now we will use these endings in sentences. Jump on the word or syllable in **boldface** type. Look for and use ligatures and blends.

1. The sun shines almost **e**very day.

2. The **mail** arrives on Monday.

3. Mary swims **eight** times a week.

4. Professor Allen drives **ele**ven miles to work.

5. I gave away **all** the tickets on time.

6. We have **eggs** and potatoes every day.

7. John is **al**ways eager to please.

8. The **la**tches on the suitcases are all broken.

9. **Fred's** ties are too loud.

10. **Su**san's decision to do her homework was good.

11. The **boys'** old bikes are blue and yellow.

12. The **chil**dren's shoes are in the closet.

EXERCISE 14. Activities on the Sentences for Practice

a. **Diagramming.** Diagram the following sentences from Exercise 11. Circle the ligatures and blends.

The **chil**dren packed their bags for camp.

The **plane** landed at the airport on time.

Jim taped his photograph to the wall.

We **ska**ted at the roller skating rink yesterday.

She served **ice** cream and cake for dessert.

b. More Sentences to Diagram. Diagram the following sentences from Exercise 12. Circle the ligatures and blends.

Mary swims **eight** times a week.

Professor Allen drives **ele**ven miles to work.

We have **eggs** and potatoes every day.

The **la**tches on the suitcases are all broken.

Susan's decision to do her homework was good.

LESSON 11

Using Upward Intonation for Yes/No Questions

OBJECTIVES

In this lesson, you will learn to use appropriate intonation for questions that require a *yes* or *no* answer. These questions have a different intonation pattern from questions that ask for information (Lesson 7). You will also develop some conversational skills that can be used in a variety of situations.

Things to Remember:

■ Review Lesson 3 on average pitch. You will need this information in making yes/no questions.

■ Continue to use ligatures and blends.

INTONATION FOR ASKING YES/NO QUESTIONS

A Review of Intonation for Questions that Ask for Information

This is the pattern used in standard sentences and questions that ask for information. Diagrammed, it looks like this:

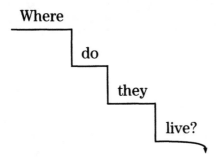

Intonation for Yes/No Questions

For questions that require a *yes* or *no* in the answer, standard intonation is *reversed*. In other words, for yes/no questions, we start low in pitch (slightly below our average pitch level) and then step *up* in pitch on each syllable to the end of the question. See *Figure 11–1*.

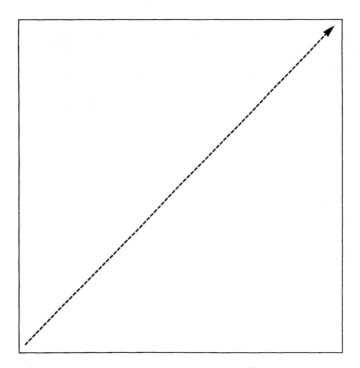

Figure 11–1. Yes/no question intonation. Reverse the intonation used for information asking questions to form standard yes/no questions.

Diagrammed, it looks like this:

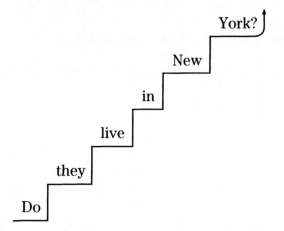

EXERCISE 1. Questions with Three Syllables

a. Using numbers instead of words, practice these two very common intonation patterns. Then practice the sentences.

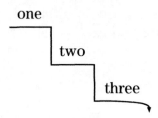

1. What are they?
2. Who knows him?
3. Why don't we?
4. Where are they?
5. When is it?

b. Reverse the pattern in Exercise 1a to produce yes/no questions.

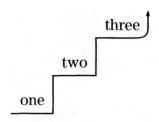

1. Is he there?
2. Will she wait?
3. May I stay?
4. Should Jane call?

5. Are you late?
6. Does it work?
7. Can you go?
8. Did he write?

EXERCISE 2. Questions with Four Syllables

a. In this set of exercises, we will use four syllables.

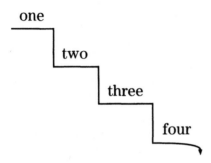

1. Why is he here?
2. When is the class?
3. Whose car is it?
4. Where are my keys?
5. Who's leaving now?

b. Reverse the pattern in Exercise 2a to produce yes/no questions.

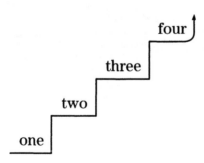

1. Will you wait here?
2. Is that your friend?
3. Do you want tea?
4. Did you leave this?
5. Are they leaving?
6. Should you do that?
7. May I help you?
8. Can you play golf?

EXERCISE 3. Questions with Six Syllables

a. In this set, sentence length has been increased to six syllables to help in obtaining greater control of this pattern.

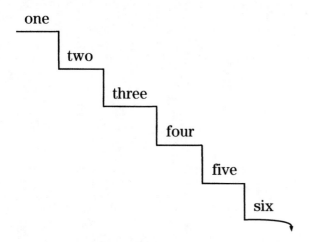

1. What is your new address?
2. When did your mother call?
3. Where is my plane ticket?
4. Whose baseball glove is this?
5. How much is a movie?

b. Now reverse the pattern shown in Exercise 3a for these yes/no questions.

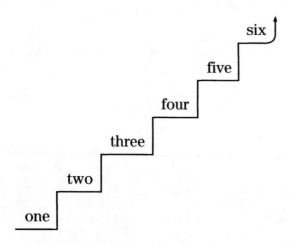

1. Is he coming for lunch?
2. Are they waiting for us?
3. Did my advisor call?
4. Will you please take this book?
5. Do you like chocolate cake? (Pronounce *choc'late* with two syllables)
6. Could you open the door?

7. Should we wait for the bus?
8. Am I saying it right?

EXERCISE 4. Diagramming Information and Yes/No Questions

Diagram these sentences as appropriate. Practice what you have diagrammed. Remember to use ligatures and blends.

1. Where are you planning to spend your vacation?

2. Are you thinking of going to Madrid?

3. Can you travel during the holidays?

4. Whose luggage was left in the airport?

5. Will they remember to take the tickets?

6. How will you get to the airport?

EXERCISE 5. Playing the Game: *Who am I?* with Yes/No Questions

You will be given the name of a famous person and will answer yes/no questions until the identity of the person is guessed correctly.

> **Example:** The name selected is *Mahatma Gandhi* (not known by others playing the game)
>
> Question 1: *Are you a female?*   Answer: *No.*
>
> Question 2: *Are you alive?*   Answer: *No.*
>
> Question 3: *Were you a leader?*   Answer: *Yes.*
>
> The game continues until . . .
>
> Last Question: *Are you Mahatma Gandhi?*   Answer: *Yes.*
>
> The person guessing the identity of the person correctly becomes "it" for the next round.

MAKING CONVERSATION

People don't always talk about important things. Many times they just want to share ideas about very common topics. When a person has the art of "making conversation," that person is considered interesting and friendly, and as a result, others enjoy the company of a good conversationalist.

The ability to make conversation, talking about interesting but relatively common topics, is important to you as a communicator and as a speaker of American English. You need to develop this ability because it will (a) help other people to get to know you and help you to know them; (b) make you more relaxed around others; (c) improve your ability to interact socially; and (d) give you some excellent opportunities to use and learn more about American English and its culture.

What do people talk about when they make conversation? What are these relatively unimportant topics that we talk about all the time? Here are some examples:

The Weather	Weekend Activities
Education/School	Entertainment
Food	Sports
Work	Travel

EXERCISE 6. Writing Questions for Conversation

For each topic area two questions are given. Write four more—two information questions and two yes/no questions. Then practice the questions, using standard *jump, step, fall* intonation (there is no need for the *walk* on average pitch before the jump) for information questions, and *start low and step up in pitch on each syllable* intonation for yes/no questions. Remember to use the questions you have studied in this lesson with your classmates, colleagues, friends, and strangers. Memorize the questions that are of greatest value to you.

a. The Weather: Did you hear a weather report today?
How much rain did we get?

_____

_____

_____

_____

b. Education/School: Where's the library?
Do you study in the library?

_____

_____

_____

_____

c. Food: Where's a good restaurant?
Do you like spinach?

_____

_____

_____

_____

d. Work: Do you have a full-time job?
Where do you work?

_____

_____

_____

e. Weekend Activities: Do you have any plans for this weekend?
What are your plans for this weekend?

_____

_____

_____

f. Entertainment: Have you seen any good movies lately?
What movies have you seen?

_____

_____

_____

g. Sports: What sports do you like?
Is soccer popular in this country?

_____

_____

_____

_____

h. Travel: Do you like to travel?
Where did you go on your vacation?

_____

_____

_____

_____

EXERCISE 7. Role-playing

Here are some familiar situations. With another person, make conversation that would be appropriate in these contexts. Ask four or five questions (either yes/no or information-asking), possibly taken from Exercise 6. Provide suitable answers.

Talking about your plans for a picnic. (weather)
Waiting for a class to start. (education/school)
Making plans to go out for lunch. (food)
Talking about your plans after you graduate. (work)
Talking to a colleague at work on Monday. (weekend activities)
Waiting in line for a movie. (entertainment)
Waiting for a sports event to start. (sports)
Meeting someone in a travel agency. (travel)

EXERCISE 8. Making Conversation: New Topics

With another person, make conversation related to these topics: _Family, Hobbies, Health,_ and _Current Events from the Newspaper._ Think of and ask information and yes/no questions. For the answers, walk to an important word and jump in pitch on it. Then step down to the last syllable and fall.

SOUND ADVICE

The Pronunciation of Present and Past Tense Word Endings

In previous lessons we studied use of singular "-s" and past time "-ed" word endings in both words and sentences. Now we will practice these word endings in the context of dialogs. As in the past, remember to jump in pitch on the word or syllable in **boldface** type.

Dialog 1: Cars, Ditches, and Tickets

Person 1:   Hel**lo**. Is this Rich's Car **Sales?**

Person 2:   **That's** right. **How** may I help you?

Person 1:   My **friend** needs to buy a new car. Do you sell new **cars**?

Person 2:   We sell **new** cars and trucks. Our company **also** takes trade-ins. **What's** wrong with your friend's old car?

Person 1:   **Nothing's** wrong with it. It **seems** to like ditches. **Every** time he goes for a drive, his **car** ends up in a ditch. **Some**times it crashes into fences. He **al**ready has five tickets.

Person 2:   That's an **int**eresting series of problems. **How** does he think a different car will help?

Person 1:   He thinks that **new** cars drive better.

Person 2:   Be**fore** he gets another car, **may**be he should enroll in driver's education.

Person 1:   That was the **ju**dge's idea, too. However, my **friend** thinks a new car would be **less** expensive. **Thanks** for the idea.

Dialog 2: They **Wan**ted a New Computer

Person 1:   My **fa**mily purchased a new computer. It ar**rived** yesterday.

Person 2:   **I** ordered one last week. They **have**n't delivered it yet.

Person 1:   **Tell** me how you decided which computer to get.

Person 2:   I **looked** in the newspaper and **called** computer stores. That helped a **litt**le. **What** helped you?

Person 1:   I **talked** to Tom who worked in a com**pu**ter store. He recommended a **Mac**. **Oth**ers suggested a PC. However, it was **more** complicated than I realized.

Person 2: The **more** I looked for answers, the **more** confused I became. I **fi**nally decided what to do. I **closed** my eyes and pointed to **one** of the computers in a newspaper ad.

Person 1: So you **were**n't confused or frustrated. You **sim**ply ordered the computer you **selec**ted at random.

Person 2: **Not** exactly. The **one** I pointed to would've **bankr**upted me.

Person 1: **What** did you do?

Person 2: I **closed** my eyes and pointed until I **found** one I could afford.

LESSON 12

Using Special Emphasis Intonation

OBJECTIVE

In this lesson, you will learn about a variation of standard intonation known as *special emphasis*. You will also learn a strategy to use when others do not understand you.

SPECIAL EMPHASIS INTONATION

Special emphasis is a variation of standard intonation that allows us to use the pitch jump to emphasize any important word in the sentence. Words that contribute to the topic of the conversation are important. For this reason, the word that you select for the pitch jump will usually gain its importance from something that has been said before in the conversation. In special emphasis

- The word you jump on should be very important to your message, and

- As with standard intonation, pitch is used instead of loudness.

To see how special emphasis intonation works, repeat the following sentences, jumping in pitch on the word or syllable written in **boldface** type. Although you do not change any of the words in the sentence, notice that the meaning of the sentence changes as you jump in pitch on the various words, or on the prominent syllables of these words.

John **did**n't have pizza for lunch yesterday. (standard intonation)

John didn't have pizza for lunch yesterday. (emphasizes *who*)

John didn't have **pizza** for lunch yesterday. (emphasizes *what*)

John didn't have pizza for **lunch** yesterday. (emphasizes *which meal*)

John didn't have pizza for lunch **yes**terday. (emphasizes *when*)

John didn't **have** pizza for lunch yesterday. (emphasizes that John had *something else*)

EXERCISE 1. Varying the Pitch Jump for Special Emphasis

Some of the sentences in this exercise are the same ones that were used for practice in Lesson 10. Now, however, the pitch jump will change to reflect a different (special) emphasis from *standard intonation*. Say each sentence aloud until you are able to make each intended change correctly and automatically. Remember to include all ligatures and blends. The word or syllable usually selected for the pitch jump in standard intonation is in **bold**.

Example: Ray **won't** type his manuscript. (standard intonation)

Ray (not Tom)	**Ray** won't type his manuscript.
type (not write)	Ray won't **type** his manuscript.
his (not her)	Ray won't type **his** manuscript.
manuscript (not book)	Ray won't type his **ma**nuscript.

1. He **asked** us a few other questions.

   few (but not all)
   us (but not them)
   questions (but not requests)

2. **Sal**ly is driving her car to Arizona.

   driving (but not towing)
   her (but not John's)
   car (but not truck)
   Arizona (not Colorado)

3. **Who** put the keys under the desk?

   keys (not books)
   desk (not table)
   under (not on)

4. He wants **no** part in our plan.

   He (not you)
   plan (not project)
   wants (not desires)

5. **Sue** read novels in her English class.

   novels (not poems)
   read (not wrote)
   English (not Spanish)
   her (not our)

6. **Pam** and her sister took the same anatomy class.

   sister (not brother)
   same (not different)
   anatomy (not physics)

7. **How** old is the administration building?

   old (not new)
   administration (not science)

8. I am **an**xious to be on her thesis committee.

   I (not you)
   her (not his)
   thesis (not dissertation)

9. Sam walks **three** miles to work everyday.

    Sam (not George)
    walks (not jogs)
    miles (not blocks)
    work (not school)
    everyday (not just yesterday)

10. I **wan**ted to thank him for all he did on Monday.

    I (not Mary)
    thank (not scold)
    him (not her)
    all (not a part of what he did)

EXERCISE 2. A Story for Special Emphasis Practice

In this story, underline all pitch jumps. Use either special emphasis or standard intonation to convey the interpretation *you* want. Although a variety of words may be selected for the pitch jump, do not jump too many times within the same sentence. Circle all ligatures and blends. Prepare to read your interpretation aloud.

THE BIRTHDAY PARTY

Who was going to have the best birthday ever? Pam was. Excitement was everywhere. We baked a wonderful cake. Pam opened her gifts. She was very happy with her treasures. "Give Pam some cake," someone said. I picked up the cake. Bill said, "Don't give Pam all the cake. Give Pam some cake." I started to give everyone a piece of the cake. "No," said Alice, "Give Pam some cake." Pretending that I was confused, I asked, "Why should I give Pam some cake? Why don't you give Pam some cake?" It was still a very happy party. The cake was delicious. Pam had more cake than anybody.

EXERCISE 3. Comic Strip Presentation

Each person will obtain a different comic strip of at least 5 pictures (frames) from a Sunday newspaper. *Blondie* works particularly well. We will prepare these miniature stories for oral presentation.

a. Read the comic strip and write down any new words that you need to learn to pronounce.

b. Decide where you will jump in each sentence of the dialog and mark these places. Your teacher will help you with sentences that are long. Remember the patterns you need to use for questions and special emphasis.

c. Prepare to present your comic strip.

■ Prepare a short introduction for the comic strip.

■ Introduce each picture (or frame) in sequence, including any explanations or transitions that you need.

■ Be sure to plan where to jump in your introduction and transition sentences, including any special emphases that you want to make.

Example *(with possible jumps in **boldface** type)*: "In this comic strip, **Blon**die is preparing dinner. The **Bum**steads have invited the Woodleys to dinner. Blondie is making spa**ghet**ti. In the **first** picture, she is alone in the kitchen. She says, I **think** this needs more garlic."

d. Present your comic strip.

A STRATEGY FOR MAKING YOURSELF UNDERSTOOD

Frequently, we say something that our listener does not understand. What can we do? Here is a strategy that you can use when this situation occurs.

1. Control your emotions because there are many reasons why people may not understand.

2. Repeat what you just said.
   a. You probably forgot to use correct intonation.
   b. Use *walk, jump, step, fall.*
   c. Repeat the most important part of what you just said.

3. Think about ways to speak more clearly.
   a. Slow down syllable rate.
   b. Pause before or after important words.
   c. Use ligatures and blends.
   d. Pronounce the ends of words.
   e. Make sure that your grammar is correct.

4. Repair the part of the sentence that your listener did not understand.

    a. Pronounce the missed word in standard intonation.

    b. Spell new or difficult words for your listener.

        (1) Learn the letters of the alphabet.

        (2) Jump on the first letter and step down on each syllable after that, with a fall at the end.

5. Change your message.

    a. Select words that are easier to understand.

    b. Use shorter sentences.

EXERCISE 4. Role-playing

Two people will make up a dialog for one or more of these situations. Each person should speak at least six times. Be sure to practice what you have learned, including special emphasis intonation and the strategy for making yourself understood.

Situation 1

You broke your arm. The doctor needs some information to know how to treat you. Discuss your accident with the doctor.

Situation 2

You need to speak to your advisor in order to drop a class. Your advisor wants to find out why you are dropping the class at this late date.

Situation 3

You saw your best friend having dinner in a restaurant with *your* "special someone." You need to find out why. Explore this situation with your friend.

Situation 4

You borrowed your friend's brand new sports car but you had an accident. Now you have to tell your friend about the accident. The owner of the fancy car might not like your report.

Situation 5

You haven't had an increase in salary since you started working at this company three years ago. You go to the office to ask your employer for a raise.

Situation 6

You have two invitations for dinner for the same evening. Although you would like to accept both invitations, you can't. You go to visit one of the persons who invited you to work out the problem.

Situation 7

You have been overcharged by $20 for your textbooks at the bookstore. You go to the bookstore to discuss the matter with the cashier who sold you the books.

Situation 8

Ask your friend for a loan of $100 in order to buy something you really need.

LESSON 13

Rhythm: Using Time in Speaking

OBJECTIVE

In this lesson, you will learn to use two important elements of rhythm in speaking: *duration* and *pauses*. Duration refers to the length of a speech sound within a syllable, usually the vowel sound of that syllable. Vowels in syllables selected for the pitch jump and final fall are lengthened. Syllables containing the neutral vowel tend to be shorter in duration. Pauses are silences that, when used appropriately, make speech more effective.

RHYTHM

In Lesson 2, we used the example of a marching band moving in step to a pattern of repeated beats, usually provided by the drums. Without rhythm the movements of the members of the band would be irregular. In fact, they would resemble a group of people walking down the street. Although every person is walking to a particular rhythm, there is no timing of movements that characterizes the entire group. Some individuals may be in a hurry, so they walk with a faster rhythm than those who are walking slowly to enjoy the scenery. Others might walk until they see something of interest; then they pause.

A particular language imposes its rhythm on everyone who speaks it. Notice that when people speak in unison, as when they recite the "pledge of allegiance" to the flag, they all speak at the same rate and with the same syllable duration. They even pause at the same time and in the same places, just like a marching band. In other words, when we speak in unison, we adhere strictly to the rhythm of the language.

Understanding Duration

You have already been using duration in speaking American English from early in this text. Remember that words like *oh* or *ah*, spoken on a sigh, are longer in length than these expressions placed within a phrase such as *Oh, no.* or *Ah, how nice.* You have also used duration on the last syllable of practically every sentence that you have spoken. The fall in pitch on the last syllable requires longer length because time is required for the final fall in pitch to occur. To understand this concept better, go back in this text to some of the sentences and dialogs that you have studied. Notice how the final fall requires more time, therefore greater duration. Notice, too, that it is the vowel that lengthens, not the consonant. It is easier to lengthen vowels. The consonants are more or less constant in duration.

You have also been using increased duration for the pitch jump in phrases and sentences. The prominent syllable of an important word is longer as well as higher in pitch than the surrounding syllables. Every time you jump in pitch, you also increase the duration of that syllable slightly.

A word of four syllables, for example, may have a *walk, jump, step, fall* intonation similar to a sentence of four one-syllable words. Compare *education* (jump on **ca**) and *I will **do** it* (jump on **do**). However, when a word is placed within a sentence, its intonation pattern will change to fit the intonation of the entire sentence. Compare *education* and *I want a **good** education*. The pitch jump no longer occurs on ca, but on **good**. What, then, happens to ca of *education*? It is lengthened more than the surrounding syllables. American English helps us to maintain durational differences by having a very short neutral vowel, /ə/, as usually found in the syllables before and after ca in *education*.

The durations in American English are very short. You have already experienced how your ear can perceive very small steps in pitch. We can also perceive small differences in duration. Therefore, the durational changes that you make do not have to be long.

EXERCISE 1. A Review of the Durational Components in *Walk, Jump, Step, Fall*

a. **Lengthening the Final Pitch Fall**. Say the following words or expressions *without* and then *with* a fall in pitch.

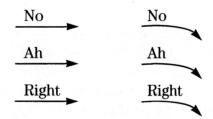

b. **Lengthening the Syllables with the Pitch Jump and Final Fall**. Repeat these sentences, jumping on the word or syllable in **boldface** type, but falling on the underlined word.

1. She **wants** to go <u>home</u>.

2. The **deaf** speak with their <u>hands</u>.

3. A**gain** and again he <u>tried</u>.

4. **Ga**ry forgot Pat's <u>lunch</u>.

5. **How** many books did the child <u>read</u>?

6. The child read **twelve** <u>books</u>.

7. We **went** to the mall to <u>shop</u>.

8. We found **ten** dollars on the <u>floor</u>.

EXERCISE 2. Using Longer Duration in Syllables Not Receiving the Pitch Jump

a. **Words Spoken Alone and in Sentences.** When a word is said by itself, the stressed syllable is higher in pitch and longer in duration than the other syllables. When used in a sentence, the pitch jump may occur on another word. Yet, the stressed syllable of the word said alone maintains its same duration although it does *not* have the pitch jump. To see how this process works, say the word in isolation, jumping on the syllable in **boldface** type. In sentence "a," the jump occurs on the same word said in isolation. In sentence "b," the jump occurs on another word, but duration, shown by the underlined word or syllable, is maintained.

1. education
   - a. An edu**ca**tion is useful.
   - b. I want a **good** edu<u>ca</u>tion.

2. **te**levision
   - a. My **te**levision set is broken.
   - b. **How** much is that <u>te</u>levision set?

3. con**tin**ue
   - a. She'll con**tin**ue the project.
   - b. She **won't** con<u>tin</u>ue the project.

4. ap**point**ment
   - a. The ap**point**ment was set for Friday.
   - b. We **set** the ap<u>point</u>ment for Friday.

5. **yes**terday
   - a. **Yes**terday we started on our trip.
   - b. We **star**ted on our trip <u>yes</u>terday.

6. pi**a**no
   - a. The pi**a**no needs tuning.
   - b. My **mo**ther plays the pi<u>a</u>no well.

7. **pho**tograph
   - a. The **pho**tograph was out of focus.
   - b. We **took** the <u>pho</u>tograph quickly.

8. ac**coun**ting
   - a. The ac**coun**ting department has many people.
   - b. My **ma**jor is ac<u>coun</u>ting.

9. de**vel**opment
   - a. Our de**vel**opment plan was accepted.
   - b. The **class** is about physical de<u>vel</u>opment.

10. engi**neer**ing
    - a. Engi**neer**ing majors are in high demand.
    - b. My e**lec**trical engi<u>neer</u>ing classes are over.

b. **Using the Pronunciation Notebook (see *Appendix C*).** Select eight (8) words that you have written in your *Pronunciation Notebook*, and write two sentences like those in Exercise 2a. In one sentence, the word you entered will have the pitch jump on its primary syllable. In the second sentence, the pitch jump will be replaced by duration. Practice saying your sentences until they are understandable.

Vowel Duration in Words Like *Lock* and *Log*

Perhaps you have been told that the difference between words like *lock* and *log* is that the final sound in *lock* is unvoiced but the /g/ in *log* is voiced. What you probably were not told was that the duration of the vowel in these two words is also different. See *Figure 13–1*. The vowel in *lock* is shorter than the vowel in *log*. If

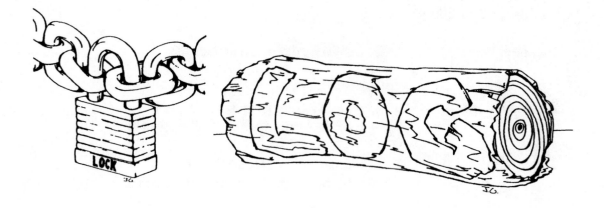

Figure 13–1. Vowel Duration. The vowel is longer in *log* than in *lock*.

you lengthen the vowel in *lock*, it may sound enough like *log* that people will not understand you. Likewise, in the words *cab* and *cap*, *bead* and *beat*, *bag* and *back*, and *ridge* and *rich*, the vowel in the first word is longer than in the second word of the pair. In fact, vowel duration may be more important than the actual voicing of final consonants.

EXERCISE 3. Words for Practice

In these words, make the vowel in the first word longer than the same vowel in the second word. Say each word with a falling pitch.

Longer Vowel Duration	Shorter Vowel Duration
rib	rip
cab	cap
cob	cop
cub	cup
ad	at
bead	beet
bud	but
grade	great
ride	right
leave	leaf
prove	proof
log	lock
bag	back
bug	buck
rag	rack
prize	price
rise	rice
buzz	bus

eyes	ice
knees	niece
fleas	fleece

EXERCISE 4. Sentences for Practice

Practice these pairs of sentences. Be sure to lengthen the vowel if the following consonant is voiced. Jump on the word written in **boldface** type.

1. a. The **prize** was three hundred dollars.
   b. The **price** was three hundred dollars.

2. a. The **cub** was little.
   b. The **cup** was little.

3. a. The **beet** was round.
   b. The **bead** was round.

4. a. The **back** was closed.
   b. The **bag** was closed.

5. a. The **cab** was yellow.
   b. The **cap** was yellow.

6. a. The **buzz** was loud.
   b. The **bus** was loud.

7. a. My **knees** will get sunburned.
   b. My **niece** will get sunburned.

8. a. **Eyes** can be cold.
   b. **Ice** can be cold.

9. a. The **fleas** went everywhere.
   b. The **fleece** went everywhere.

10. a. The **dyes** were white and black.
    b. The **dice** were white and black.

EXERCISE 5. Testing Your Progress

Read each of the sentences in Exercise 4 to someone else. Ask your listener to tell you what you said (either sentence "a" or "b"). Figure the percentage of the times you were understood correctly.

$$\frac{\text{Total Words Understood:} \underline{\hspace{2cm}}}{\text{Total Words Read:} \quad 20} \times 100 = \underline{\hspace{1.5cm}} \text{ Percent}$$

THE NEUTRAL VOWEL IN AMERICAN ENGLISH

If duration is important in American English, and we can make certain vowels longer during the pitch jump or the fall at the end of the sentence, then we also need a way to shorten vowels. When a very short vowel is needed, speakers of American English use the *schwa*, or neutral vowel, a very special kind of vowel made in the middle of the mouth (Edwards, 1992). We say that this vowel is used to *center the tone* (see Lesson 2) for American English, the general area around which American English speech is centered.

This neutral vowel, often shown phonetically as /ə/, will not usually occur in the syllable with the pitch jump. It is frequent in other syllables, however. In fact, it is our most frequently used vowel, and any vowel at times may be pronounced as the neutral vowel. In American English, the consonants are pronounced more than the vowels.

EXERCISE 6. The Neutral Vowel in Two-Syllable Words

Each of these words contains the neutral vowel. First, underline the syllable that receives the pitch jump. In this exercise, it will *never* have the schwa. Then draw a circle around the neutral vowel in the remaining syllable. Notice that these words show that the vowel letters—a, e, i, o, and u—may be pronounced as the neutral vowel. Finally, practice these words noting the central placement of the schwa.

Example: (a)while
cancel

allow	nickel	pencil
today	capsule	cola
disease	submit	pilot
reward	canal	album

EXERCISE 7. Neutral Vowels in Three Syllable Words

Underline the syllable that receives the pitch jump. Then draw a circle around all the neutral vowels. Practice pronouncing each word with appropriate intonation and pronunciation of the neutral vowel.

Example: di̲rector

banana	appraisal	mischievous
principal	develop	description
understand	attention	arena

EXERCISE 8. Neutral Vowels in Words of Several Syllables

All these words have two vowels that are not reduced. <u>Underline</u> the pitch jump and draw a circle around all neutral vowels. Not every vowel in a word can be reduced to /ə/.

Example: co̲nventional

education	democratic	confrontation
communication	segregated	independent
universal	refrigerator	participant

EXERCISE 9. Neutral Vowels in Sentences

In each sentence, <u>underline</u> the one syllable that receives the pitch jump. Then draw a circle around all neutral vowels. As usual, practice each sentence.

1. The students read the Declaration of Independence.

2. The birth of colonial North America was the result.

3. When was the North American Revolution?

USING PAUSES IN SPEECH

Nonnative speakers of a language tend to pause too many times, frequently before and after each word. Too many pauses make speech difficult to understand. However, you will not use too many pauses if you use ligatures and blends in standard intonation.

There are three kinds of pauses (Goldman-Eisler, 1968). The first is the *respiratory pause*. Native speakers pause to breathe between sentences, not in the middle of sentences. Therefore, these pauses are used to fill the lungs with air in preparation for the sentence that follows. Nonnative speakers of American English may forget to breathe between sentences. They pause to breathe between words, thus making speech irregular and difficult to understand.

The second kind of pause is the *within sentence pause*. The within sentence pause is too short to be used for breathing. It usually occurs at natural breaks between the major parts of a sentence. In writing, punctuation may signal where pauses may occur. They also are used before or after an important word that you want your listener to remember, such as the name of a person or a word taken from another language. These pauses do not interrupt intonation. They occur while using *walk, jump, step, fall* intonation. After the within sentence pause, continue the intonation pattern that you started before the pause.

Finally, there is the *hesitation pause*. These are unplanned, long pauses within or between sentences during those times when we forget a word or do not remember how to pronounce something. Nonnative speakers use more hesitation pauses than native speakers because of grammatical and vocabulary difficulties. Hesitation pauses cause irregularities in rhythm that are confusing to the listener.

EXERCISE 10. Pausing in the Story of "The Fox and the Grapes"

Mark all of the pauses in this part of the story with a slash (/).

Soon he became very tired. Worn out by his efforts, he left the vineyard. "Well,"

he muttered, "I never really wanted those grapes anyway. I'm sure they are sour.

They probably have worms in them, too!"

The moral of the story is: We might not like what we cannot easily attain.

EXERCISE 11. Review. Circle the correct answer from the words in *italics*.

1. One of the components of rhythm is *duration / loudness*.

2. The vowel sound in the word *cab* is *long / short*.

3. The vowel sound in the word *back* is *long / short*.

4. The word *banana* has *two / three* neutral vowels.

5. A respiratory pause is used to *think about what to say / breathe*.

6. A hesitation pause is used to *think about what to say / breathe*.

7. It is *appropriate / inappropriate* to pause before and after each word.

8. In determining where to use a within sentence pause, *the pitch jump / punctuation* may be helpful.

SOUND ADVICE

Avoiding Extra Syllables

As you know, syllables are very important to rhythm. Our message literally rides on the syllables we produce. If extra, meaningless syllables are added to this message, they may confuse our listener. Some students add an extra syllable when two difficult sounds occur together in speech, or they may add an unneeded syllable before a word that starts with a difficult combination such as /sp/ in *sport* or /st/ in *student*. A way to avoid using meaningless syllables is to use a *within sentence pause* before these particular sound combinations.

Some combinations of sounds are so similar or so difficult to pronounce together that speakers of American English may not pronounce all of the sounds in the combination. Although we do not recommend deleting sounds, some sounds may be deleted without affecting speech. Here we will discuss two patterns. The first is the "–nd" followed by another consonant. In the word *grandfather*, notice the "–ndf–" combination. Many speakers will delete the "d" and pronounce the word as *granfather*, a very natural pronunciation.

■ In –nd + consonant combinations, delete the /d/.

The second combination involves /t/. When /t/ occurs with a consonant before *and* after it, the /t/ may be omitted. In the phrase, *nearest bunch*, the /t/ has /s/ before and /b/ after. In pronouncing this difficult combination, many speakers of American English will delete the /t/ and say, *neares bunch*.

■ In consonant + –t– + consonant combinations, delete the /t/.

Remember, these guidelines do not apply when ligatures may be made.

EXERCISE 12. Using Pauses to Avoid Extra Syllables

In these words, test yourself to see if you add an extra syllable. Then try the phrases with a very short within sentence pause, indicated by a slash (/). As always, jump on the word or syllable printed in **boldface** type.

1. the **beach** / there
2. to **wait** / for
5. a **good** / sport
6. **two** / students
7. **is** / from
8. **Pat** / forgot
9. He was / **thir**sty.
3. have / some **time**
4. **talk** / to
10. the **card** / party
11. **just** about / famished
12. John / **still** / studies
13. an **old** / stadium
14. **wants** / them

EXERCISE 13. Deleting Sounds to Avoid Extra Syllables

Test yourself to see if you add an extra syllable in these phrases. Then say the phrases without the /d/ or /t/ in the difficult combinations. As always, jump on the word or syllable printed in **boldface** type.

1. **nea**rest bunch
2. **sun**-ripened grapes
3. **left** the vineyard
4. **learned** that
5. a **soft** color
6. **around** the corner
7. the **finest** silk
8. the **next** question
9. **waxed** paper
10. **thrift** shop
11. **jumped** for
12. the **next** chapter
13. **iced** tea
14. **packed** the bags

LESSON 14

More on the American English Syllable

OBJECTIVE

In this lesson you will learn more about:

■ the structure of the American English syllable,

■ some ways that consonants are combined into *clusters*, and

■ how to guess the pronunciaton of difficult words

AMERICAN ENGLISH SYLLABLE STRUCTURE: CLUSTERS

In Lesson 2, we learned that the unit of speech is the syllable and the basic syllable is made of a consonant followed by a vowel. All languages have syllables. Yet, not all syllables are constructed the same as in American English. In fact, many syllable combinations are permitted.

When two or more consonants are pronounced together, they form a consonant *cluster* or group. Clusters may not be as easy to pronounce as single consonants in a syllable. Clusters may occur at the beginning and end of words. Some students may have difficulty with clusters that begin words and some with clusters that end words (C = consonant, V = vowel).

The Basic Syllable:	CV	*go*
Other Single Consonant Syllables:	VC	*at*
	CVC	*sat*
Clusters that Begin Syllables:	CCV	*tree*
	CCCV	*spree*
	CCVC	*stop*
	CCCVC	*street*
Clusters that End Syllables:	VCC	*and*
	VCCC	*acts*
	CVCC	*tops*
	CVCCC	*tents*
Clusters that Begin and End Syllables:	CCVCC	*stops*
	CCCVCC	*streets*
	CCVCCC	*trusts*
	CCCVCCC	*splints*

Clusters that Begin Words

Fortunately, only a select group of letters (or sounds) may be used to form clusters at the beginning of words. Three major groups of clusters may be discussed: (1) those that end with /r/, (2) those that end with /l/, and (3) those that begin with /s/ (Heilman, 1993).

/l/ clusters: bl, cl/kl, fl, gl, pl, sl, spl

    Examples: *black, clock, flag, glove, play, slow, splash*

/r/ clusters: br, cr, dr, fr, gr, pr, tr, scr, spr, str, thr

    Examples: *brain, cry, drink, fry, green, pray, tray, scrape, spray, strap, throw*

/s/ clusters: sc/sk, sl, sm, sn, sp, st, sw, scr, spl, spr, str

   Examples: *scale/skate, slow, smile, snow, spot, stop, swing, scrape, splash, spray, strap*

EXERCISE 1. Building Words with /l/ Clusters

Make different words by adding the sounds in the second column to the beginning of the word in the first column. Then make another word by adding the sound in the fourth column to the original word. Practice saying all the words.

   Example: lack *add* /b/ *to make* = <u>black</u> ; *add* /s/ *to make* = <u>slack</u>

   lot   *add* /s/ *to make* = _____ ; *add* /p/ *to make* = _____

   late   /p/   = _____ ;   /s/   = _____

   lip   /s/   = _____ ;   /f/   = _____

   latter   /p/   = _____ ;   /f/   = _____

   lock   /c/   = _____ ;   /b/   = _____

   lay   /p/   = _____ ;   /s/   = _____

   light   /f/   = _____ ;   /s/   = _____

   low   /s/   = _____ ;   /g/   = _____

   lass   /g/   = _____ ;   /c/   = _____

   lame   /f/   = _____ ;   /b/   = _____

   lash   /c/   = _____ ;   /f/   = _____

   land   /g/   = _____ ;   /b/   = _____

EXERCISE 2. Building Words with /r/ Clusters

Make different words by adding the sounds in the second column to the beginning of the word in the first column. Then make another word by adding the sound in the fourth column to the original word. Practice saying all the words.

   Example: ray *add* /p/ *to make* = <u>pray</u> ; *add* /t/ *to make* = <u>tray</u>

   rain   /b/   = _____   /d/   = _____

room	/g/	= _____	/b/	= _____
rip	/t/	= _____	/d/	= _____
raft	/c/	= _____	/d/	= _____
rink	/d/	= _____	/b/	= _____
right	/f/	= _____	/b/	= _____
rack	/t/	= _____	/c/	= _____
rust	/c/	= _____	/t/	= _____
ride	/p/	= _____	/b/	= _____
risk	/f/	= _____	/b/	= _____
rim	/t/	= _____	/b/	= _____
race	/t/	= _____	/b/	= _____
rush	/b/	= _____	/c/	= _____

Exercise 3. Building Words with /s/ Clusters. Make different words by adding the /s/ sound to the beginning of the word provided. Then practice the original word and the different word with the beginning /s/ cluster.

Example: mile *add* /s/ *to make* = <u>smile</u>

pot	*add* /s/ to *make*	= _____
top	/s/	= _____
care	/s/	= _____
mall	/s/	= _____
mother	/s/	= _____
nail	/s/	= _____
table	/s/	= _____
team	/s/	= _____

topping	/s/	= _____
wear	/s/	= _____
wing	/s/	= _____
car	/s/	= _____

EXERCISE 4. Building Words with Three-Sound Clusters: str, scr, spl, spr

Take the word that is given in the first column. Then add the sound in the second column to produce a different word. Finally, add the last sound to this word to form a three-sound cluster.

Example: rap *add* /t/ = <u>trap</u> *then add* /s/ *to make* = <u>strap</u>

rain *add*   /t/ = _____ *then add* /s/ *to make* = _____

latter	/p/ = _____	+	/s/	= _____
rip	/t/ = _____	+	/s/	= _____
lay	/p/ = _____	+	/s/	= _____
ray	/p/ = _____	+	/s/	= _____
rapping	/t/ = _____	+	/s/	= _____
ream	/c/ = _____	+	/s/	= _____
ray	/t/ = _____	+	/s/	= _____
roll	/t/ = _____	+	/s/	= _____
ripe	/t/ = _____	+	/s/	= _____

Consonant Clusters that End Words

The ends of words are very important in American English and are usually pronounced. They carry more grammatical information than the beginnings of words. If you do not pronounce the ends of words, speech will be difficult to understand.

Clusters that commonly end words may be grouped in a manner similar to clusters that begin words. As we have already seen in other lessons (8, 9, and 10, in particular), "s" to indicate plurals, possessives, and present time (pronounced /s/ or /z/), and "ed" for past time (pronounced /t/ or /d/) may be added to the ends of words. The result of this action is frequently a consonant cluster *(walks, cooked)*. Because these word endings were practiced before, they will not be covered again in this lesson.

/s, z/ clusters—for plurals, possessives, and present time

> **Examples**: *cats, dogs, cat's, dog's, walks, runs* (See Lessons 8 and 10 for practice material)

/t, d/ clusters—for past tense

> **Examples**: *walked, begged* (See Lessons 9 and 10 for practice material)

There are three other groups of end of word clusters: (1) those that begin with /s/, (2) those that begin with /l/, and (3) those that begin with one of the nasal consonants, /m/, /n/ or /ng/.

/s/ clusters: /sp/, /st/, /sk/

> **Examples**: *crisp, list, desk*

/l/ clusters: /ld/, /lf/, /lk/, /lm/, /lth/, /lp/, /ls/, /lt/, /lv/

> **Examples**: *child, self, milk, film, wealth, help, else, adult, twelve*

/n, ng/ or /m/ clusters: /nd/, /nth/, /ngk/, /nj/, /nch/, /nts/, /mp/

> **Examples**: *band, month, think, change, inch, dance, camp*

> ***Pronunciation Note:*** In the word *think*, the "nk" combination is pronounced /ngk/. Other examples are *drink, sink, pink*, and *ink*. The combinations "nts," "nse," and "nce" at the ends of words are pronounced /nts/ as in *cents, dense*, and *dance*.

EXERCISE 5. Words that End with /s/ Clusters

The /s/ sound is very productive in American English. In addition to helping to form plurals, possessives, and to mark verbs for present tense, it is also used with several consonants to form words. Pronounce these words, making sure that you are pronouncing the final consonant clusters. Remember to jump *and* fall in pitch on the words of one syllable. For words of more than one syllable, jump on the syllable written in **boldface** type.

wasp	clasp	lisp	crisp	gro**tesque**
grasp	most	must	frost	coast
almost	as**sist**	**August**	in**sist**	**sma**llest
sug**gest**	mask	gasp	desk	disk
dust	**as**terisk	brisk	task	pictur**esque**

EXERCISE 6. Words that End with /l/ Clusters

The /l/ clusters are also frequent in American English. Notice all the consonants that may be combined with /l/ to form common words. Pronounce these words, making sure that you are pronouncing the final consonant clusters.

build	child	field	cold	mild
old	with**hold**	**bill**fold	shelf	self
golf	my**self**	her**self**	elf	milk
silk	elk	film	elm	realm
help	scalp	pulp	else	pulse
false	**im**pulse	belt	fault	guilt
melt	salt	**adult**	**as**phalt	re**sult**
difficult	health	wealth	dis**solve**	twelve
in**volve**	valve	solve	re**volve**	e**volve**

EXERCISE 7. Words that End with /n, ng/ or /m/ Clusters

The nasal sounds may also combine with some consonants to form common words. Pronounce these words, making sure that you are pronouncing the final consonant clusters completely.

ground	hand	blend	find	fund
be**hind**	**dia**mond	under**stand**	**second**	pre**tend**
chance	dance	fence	rinse	since
tense	**ba**lance	an**nounce**	ap**pear**ance	pro**nounce**
ant	don't	mint	**dis**count	paint
ap**point**	cement	a**part**ment	**mon**ument	ex**per**iment
month	ninth	el**ev**enth	**seventh**	bank
drink	ink	sink	tank	trunk
inch	branch	bunch	lunch	wrench
bench	bump	clamp	dump	jump
change	lounge	hinge	ar**range**	strange

EXERCISE 8. The Effect of Ligatures on Consonant Clusters

Ligatures often cause consonant clusters to separate so that all or part of the cluster might move to the beginning of the next word. In these sentences, circle all of the ligatures. Jump in pitch on the word or syllable in **boldface** type.

1. **Milk** is good for you.

2. **Put** the list on the desk.

3. I like **one** lump of sugar in my coffee.

4. An **inch** is longer than a centimeter.

5. We **want** to develop self esteem.

6. There are **twelve** apples left on the tree.

7. The wasp is a **dang**erous insect.

8. Change is **al**ways difficult

SOUND ADVICE

Guessing the Pronunciation of Words from Their Spelling

English, as you know, is not always pronounced as it is spelled. This feature of English spelling creates problems for native and nonnative speakers alike. We all have to learn how to pronounce (and spell) words like *enough, dough, answer, cupboard,* and *hiccough.* For these and other words, you have set up a *Pronunciation Notebook* in which to write all of the words that you need to know how to pronounce correctly. However, there are some spelling principles that we will provide, that may help in pronouncing many words with unusual spellings (Heilman, 1993).

1. **"g"**
   - sounds like /j/ when followed by i, e, or y (*giant, gem, biology*)
   - at other times, it sounds like /g/ (*game, again*)
   - is silent in combination with "ng" if the preceding part of the word is an actual word; otherwise, the /g/ is pronounced (silent: *banging, wringer*; pronounced: *angle, finger*)

2. **"c"**
   - sounds like /s/ when followed by i, e, or y (*city, cent, cycle*)
   - at other times, it sounds like /k/ (*car, across*)

3. **"x"**
   - sounds like /ks/ (*box, fox*)

4. **Silent Final "e" at the End of a Word**
   - the preceding vowel usually sounds like the alphabet letter name (*cake, fine*)

5. Letter Combinations

- ■ "ck" sounds like /k/ (*back, chicken*)
- ■ "ph" sounds like /f/ (*graph, elephant*)
- ■ "qu" sounds like /kw/ (*quick, equal*)
- ■ "le" at the end of a word, is pronounced "el" (*able, apple*)
- ■ "tion" at the end of a word, sounds like /shən/ (*election, separation*)
- ■ "ture" at the end of a word, sounds like "chure" (*picture, lecture, furniture*)

6. Silent Letters in Combinations

- ■ "wr" sounds like /r/ (*write, wrap*)
- ■ "kn/gn" sound like /n/ (*knight, gnat*)
- ■ "ps" at the start of a word, sounds like /s/ (*psychic, pseudo*)
- ■ "mb" at the end of a word, sounds like /m/ (*bomb, thumb*)

EXERCISE 9. Applying these Spelling Principles

Notice that each spelling principle above is numbered (1–6). In the space provided, write the number of all the principles that apply to these words.

Example: <u>1,4</u> gave ("g" and "silent-e")

____ comb	____ lamb	____ hanger	____ singer
____ ringing	____ condition	____ angel	____ pasture
____ necessary	____ exercise	____ geography	____ education
____ philosophy	____ sign	____ psychology	____ uncle
____ wrong	____ administration	____ knife	____ quack
____ jungle	____ appendix	____ contemplate	____ agency
____ wrecker	____ English	____ creature	____ certain

EXERCISE 10. Using Your Dictionary

At times, there are no easy rules to assist us in pronouncing words. It then becomes necessary to check the word in a dictionary and enter it in your *Pronunciation Notebook*. Here are some words that are not pronounced as they are spelled. Look them up in your dictionary and write the dictionary pronunciation on the line following each word.

rough _____   muscle _____   luscious _____

hiccough _____   special _____   ache _____

chaos _____   charade _____   says _____

handkerchief _____   orchid _____   through _____

rhythm _____   routine _____   dough _____

EXERCISE 11. Silent Syllables

Some three syllable words that have the pitch jump on the *first* syllable, have a silent *second* syllable. They actually lose a syllable. In the following words, circle the silent syllable (or vowel). Remember to jump on the first syllable as you practice these words.

Example: fam(i)ly   di(a)mond

probably   evening   grocery   nursery

chocolate   conference   every   several

interest   business   funeral   general

Some longer words also lose a syllable. Practice saying these words without the shaded syllable. Remember to jump in pitch on the syllable in **boldface** type.

vegetable   **lab**oratory   **tem**perature   di**rec**tory

LESSON 15

Intonation in Longer Sentences

OBJECTIVE

In this lesson, you will learn some simple variations of standard *walk, jump, step, fall* intonation, such as when sentences are combined or contain lists. When sentences are short and contain one important thought or idea, they usually have only one pitch jump. When sentences are long, they will usually contain more than one idea, and can have more than one pitch jump.

MAKING SENTENCES LONGER
BY ADDING ANOTHER THOUGHT

Many sentences contain more than one main thought. In other words, it is possible to have two or more sentences in one longer sentence. Look at these examples:

a. Sue likes little green apples.

b. Fred enjoys juicy oranges.

c. Sue likes little green apples and Fred enjoys juicy oranges.
Sue likes little green apples but Fred enjoys juicy oranges.

The two thoughts are used in the sentences in "c." We can jump on both **Sue** and **Fred** and then step down to the final fall on *oranges*. When two sentences are joined together with words such as *and, but, so,* or *or,* then *both* sentences may have a separate pitch jump. In the example:

I had an appointment on Friday, but I couldn't go.

there is a pitch jump on **had** and *another* on the first syllable of **could**n't.

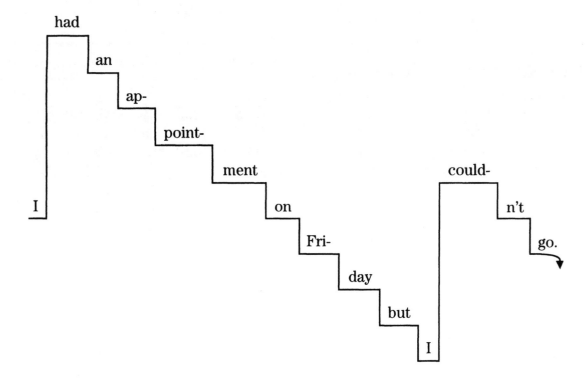

Look at this diagram carefully. As you have already seen, there are two pitch jumps, one on **had** and the other on **could**. A separate pitch jump occurs in *each* thought or idea expressed in the longer sentence. Notice that there is no final fall on *day* in *Friday*. We haven't finished the sentence and we want our listener to know that more is coming. Therefore, we continue to step down on every syllable until the next pitch jump occurs. In the first thought (*I had an appointment on Friday*), continue stepping down, even on *but I* of the second thought (*I couldn't go*). That is, step down on *an appointment on Friday, but I*, with *I* being lower in pitch than the last syllable of *Friday*. This will be followed by the second pitch jump on **could**. The usual final fall in pitch occurs on *go*. In the exercises for this lesson, remember to continue stepping down in pitch until you jump again. Then step down from that point to the final pitch fall. The final fall at the end of the sentence tells your listener that you are finished with the two-thought sentence.

DECIDING WHERE TO JUMP IN LONGER SENTENCES

Jump on Words that Contrast

In Lesson 8, we listed the kinds of words with a high probability of receiving the pitch jump. In longer sentences, the same word classes will also receive the pitch jump. In addition, words that contrast in different thoughts within the same longer sentence may *both* receive a pitch jump: **Mary** is a friend of the family, but **Bill** isn't. **John** went to Dallas on business and **Mary** met him there. **This** is good, but **that's** better. Contrasting words will usually be of the same grammatical class. For example, a noun will contrast with another noun (*John/Mary*) or two verbs may contrast, and so on.

EXERCISE 1. Contrasting Words

Here are longer sentences with contrasts. First, draw a line between the two sentences expressed in each longer sentence. Then jump in pitch on the two contrasts that are suggested. Step down in pitch between the contrasting words. Fall on the last syllable of the sentence.

> **Example:** **Mary** planned to go to a movie / but her **friend** wanted to watch television. (Contrast *Mary* and *friend*)

1. Mr. Smith wanted to stay home but his children wanted to take a vacation. (contrast *Mr.* and *children*)

2. This biology class works hard but that one works even harder. (contrast *This* and *that*)

3. Mary wanted to go to the department store so Fran took her. (*Mary/Fran*)

4. Peggy did all of her homework and Sue watched a movie on television. (*Peggy/Sue*)

5. People like to eat sweet desserts but they don't want to get fat. (contrast the verbs *like/don't*)

6. He'd like to take a vacation but he doesn't have the time. (*like/doesn't*)

7. Jim washed the dinner dishes and Julie dried them. (*Jim/Julie*)

8. I forgot to bring enough money so I'll have to borrow some. (*forgot/have*)

Jump on Words Expressing New Information

In longer sentences standard intonation is used for the first thought, with the pitch jump occurring on the new information in the second thought or idea. Contrasting words (as in Exercise 1) will usually be of the same grammatical class, but new information may be expressed in words that are not of the same class. For example, in the sentence, **John** *went to Dallas on business but he for**got** his briefcase*, we can jump on **John** (noun) and again on the second syllable of *for**got*** (verb).

EXERCISE 2. New Information

In these sentences, we will jump on the new information.

> **Example**: Mary is a **Cer**tified Public Accountant but she **can't** do her own taxes. (*Certified/can't*)

1. Jane went to the store, so she could buy some more apples.(*Jane/buy*)

2. We were on our way to the theater and the car ran out of gas. (*We/car*)

3. Mr. Fox was just about famished so he crept into a vineyard. (*just/crept*)

4. I'd like to learn several other languages but I'm too busy. (*like/too*)

5. You could ride your bike to work but the tires are flat. (*ride/tires*)

6. The children were playing in the park when a big ice cream truck came into view. (*children/big*)

7. It was time for us to leave but the baby sitter hadn't arrived yet. (*time/baby sitter*)

8. We were looking through an old book and a twenty-dollar bill fell to the floor. (*looking/twenty*)

WORDS USED TO CONNECT LONGER SENTENCES

In addition to *and, but, so,* or *or,* there are other words used to connect thoughts in longer sentences. For example, *when, if, even though, although, because, while, after,* and so on may also work in this way. Many of these two-thought sentences also have more than one pitch jump. One possible difference between these sentences and the ones joined with *and, but, so,* and *or* is that one of the pitch jumps may occur on the word that connects. These adverbs are high probability words for the pitch jump in American English.

Example: We **ce**lebrated the victory **af**ter the team won the ball game.

The most important word in the first thought is *celebrated.* We jump on the first syllable of <u>celebrated</u> and step down to the last syllable of *victory.* Then we may jump again on **after,** stepping down until we fall in pitch on the last syllable *game.*

> **Pronunciation Note:** If special emphasis is used, we may jump on any other important words in this combined sentence. For example, practice jumping on **victory** and **ball.**

EXERCISE 3. Using Other Connectives

In these sentences, first draw a line between the two main ideas. Then practice the sentences, jumping on the suggested words. Notice that these sentences contain contrasting ideas and new information. They usually contrast when the words selected for the pitch jump are of the same grammatical class, but for new information, the words may be from different classes.

Example: We **ce**lebrated the victory / **af**ter the team won the ball game.

1. After I see the play, I'll know if it's worth the money. (*after/know*)

2. When the phone finally rang, it was the wrong number. (*phone/wrong*)

3. If you write him a letter, he might answer within a week or two. (*write/might*)

4. Even though he won the lottery, he still wasn't very happy. (*Even/still*)

5. She bought a brand new car although she didn't know how to drive it. (*brand/didn't*)

6. He went to the emergency room because he was very sick. (*went/very*)

7. I'll invite her to the birthday party even though she isn't very friendly. (*invite/isn't*)

8. We'll have time to discuss our vacation plans when you get here. (*time/when*)

9. We had to leave the concert while the orchestra was playing our favorite song. (*had/orchestra*)

10. When the snows of winter have ended, we'll plan our vacation to Alaska. (*snows/plan*)

EXERCISE 4. Diagramming

Select 5 of the above sentences and diagram them showing appropriate *walk*, *jump*, *step*, and *fall* intonation.

1.

2.

3.

4.

5.

EXERCISE 5. Making Sentences

Combine these short sentences into one longer sentence by selecting an appropriate connecting word from the list. Jump in pitch twice in each combined sentence. **Select from these connecting words:** *even though, when, because, if, although, while, before, after*

Example: George jogs every day   He wants to be healthy

George jogs every day because he **wants** to be healthy.

1. We won't go to the baseball game.   It's raining very hard.

2. They're going to get married in June.   They're not in love.

3. The Smiths want to buy a house in the suburbs.   They get a loan from the bank.

4. We're going to go to the movie tomorrow.   We really don't have time tonight.

5. I'm going to enroll in Anthropology 100.   I'll take Anthropology 200.

6. John broke his leg in the accident.   No one else was hurt.

7. The students won't graduate this semester.   They don't have enough hours.

8. We have to take the test tomorrow afternoon.   We are not prepared.

9. The children will visit Disneyworld.   They visit Epcot.

10. We arrived at the airport late.   We had forgotten to pick up the tickets.

11. We need to wash the breakfast dishes.   We watch cartoons on TV.

12. I have an interview with Multinational Incorporated.   I graduate from the university.

EXERCISE 6. Diagramming

Select 5 of the sentence combinations in Exercise 5 and diagram them showing appropriate *walk, jump, step, and fall* intonation.

1.

2.

3.

4.

5.

LIST INTONATION

Frequently, we want to provide our listener with a list of persons, places, or things. For this kind of longer sentence, we will change the use of *walk, jump, step, and fall*. This slight adjustment is called *list intonation*. It is appropriate to jump on the first item in the list, but do not step down until you have said the entire item. Then step down on the second item in the list, staying on that pitch step until you have said the entire item. Continue in this manner until you get to the last item in the list. Then step down on each syllable and fall on the last syllable. Although this adjustment might seem difficult, it is very efficient because you use only one pitch step on each item, using usual step down and fall on the last item. The downward fall in pitch at the end, says, "I'm finished with this list."

Example:

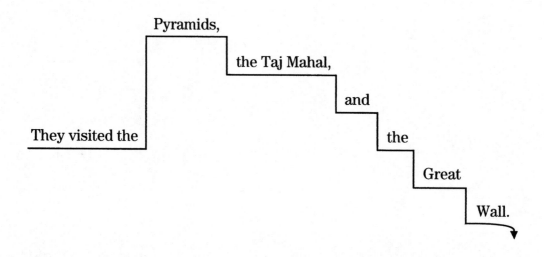

EXERCISE 7. List Intonation

Practice these sentences that use list intonation. The pitch jump is written in **boldface** type. Remember to say the entire word on the pitch jump.

1. They wanted a **house**, a car, and a boat.

2. For the party we had **cake**, punch, and cookies.

3. When camping you'll need a **tent**, a cot, and a sleeping bag.

4. The university offers a **bachelor's**, a master's, and a doctor's degree.

5. We plan to visit **Delaware**, Maryland, and Virginia.

6. You can buy **blackberries**, blueberries, raspberries, and strawberries.

7. I want a **sweater**, a computer, and a watch for my birthday.

8. Our school has **baseball**, football, soccer, and bowling teams.

9. You'll need a **dictionary**, an encyclopedia, and a thesaurus for your term paper.

10. At **two-thousand**, four-thousand, and six-thousand miles, check the **spark plugs**, the air conditioner, and the transmission.

EXERCISE 8. Making Sentences with List Intonation

From this list of words, make appropriate sentences in which you use list intonation.

Example: Monday   Wednesday   Friday

My tennis lesson is scheduled every **Monday**, Wednesday, and Friday.

1. motel	hotel	bed and breakfast
2. gloves	shoes	hats
3. fishing	hunting	hiking
4. violin	harp	cello
5. corn	wheat	alfalfa
6. Coca Cola	Pepsi	Seven-Up
7. calculator	notebook	tape recorder
8. New York	Las Vegas	San Francisco
9. bananas	cherries	oranges
10. algebra	sociology	accent modification

LESSON 16

Putting Our Knowledge to Work: How to Tell a Story

OBJECTIVE

In Lesson 9, we studied the story of "The Fox and the Grapes." In this lesson, we will review the strategy for preparing stories for presentation. It includes

■ Selecting and practicing all new or difficult words;

■ Deciding where and how many times to jump in pitch in each sentence;

■ Adding all ligatures and blends; and

■ Practicing until your speech is completely understandable.

TELLING A STORY

Every time we have an interesting experience, we want to tell our friends about it. We talk about vacations, trips, classes, letters that we have received, and many events in our lives or in the lives of others. In preparing to be better storytellers, we will participate in a series of activities that will teach us a strategy to use in telling about those important events in our lives. First, let's return to another of the famous fables of Aesop. Read about "The Fox and the Lion." Then do the activities that will help you to see how far you have come since Lesson 9, and perhaps what you need to continue to work on.

THE STORY OF "THE FOX AND THE LION"

EXERCISE 1. Adding a Moral to a Story

Here is another of Aesop's fables about a fox. First, read the story and then write an appropriate moral or lesson taught by the story. Next, prepare to tell this story by doing the activities in Exercises 2, 3, 4, 5, and 6 (select problem words, diagram the problem words, practice the problem words, mark pitch jumps, mark ligatures and blends, and practice for understanding).

There was a fox who had never seen a lion. One day he met a lion in the woods.

He was so frightened that he ran away. The next day he saw the mighty lion again.

This time he didn't run away even though he was still scared. The next time that

the fox saw the lion, he was no longer afraid. He went up to the lion and started

to talk to him as an old friend.

The moral of the story is _____

_____

_____

EXERCISE 2. Selecting the Difficult Words

Reread the story of "The Fox and the Lion," pausing to write down any words that you do not understand or think you will have difficulty pronouncing.

_____

_____

_____

EXERCISE 3. Diagramming Each Problem Word

Use your dictionary to check on definitions and to find the syllable that receives the pitch jump. Practice each word and diagram it below. Use your tape recorder, if possible.

EXERCISE 4. Dialog for Practicing Problem Words

Use each problem word in this dialog.

Student 1: **How** do you say the word _____? *(Student 1 selects a word from Exercise 1.)*

Student 2: _____. You say _____. *(Jump on the "word")*

Student 1: _____. I **like** the word _____.

Student 2: The **word** _____ could be useful.

(Student 2 then selects another problem word.)

EXERCISE 5. Marking Pitch Jumps

Go over the story again, underlining all pitch jumps (as in Lesson 9).

EXERCISE 6. Marking Ligatures and Blends

Now, circle all the ligatures and blends (as in Lesson 10).

EXERCISE 7. Telling the Story

When you have practiced sufficiently, tell the story of "The Fox and the Lion" as you have prepared it in the previous exercises.

THE STORY OF "THE TWO POTS"

EXERCISE 8. Completing a Story

Continue the strategy as with the other two stories. This time, you will complete the story *and* add the final moral just as Aesop did many years ago.

Two pots that had been used for cooking soup were carried away in a flood. One

of the pots was of finest clay and was very fragile. The other pot was of brass, a

durable metal of great strength. The pots were swept down the raging river in the

flood. The brass pot promised to protect the clay pot if the two of them would

stay together. The clay pot thanked the brass pot for the offer, but said, "_____

_____

_____

_____

_____ "

The moral of the story is: _____

_____

_____

EXERCISE 9. Writing Your Own Aesop's Fable

Using the information that is provided below, write a fable. Don't forget to use the strategy that you have learned in this lesson for telling a story.

Title: *The Bird and the Pitcher*

The Situation: The bird is very thirsty and wants a drink.
The pitcher is very narrow and deep.
It has some water at the bottom.
The bird cannot reach the water and he is too weak to break the pitcher or turn it over.
Many small stones are near the pitcher.

The Story:

Who is this story about? _____

_____

What problems does the bird have? _____

_____

_____

_____

What did the bird do? _____

_____

_____

_____

What is the moral of this story? _____

_____

_____

THE STORY OF "THE LION AND THE MOUSE"

EXERCISE 10. Using a Strategy for Telling a Story

Here is another story adapted from a fable by Aesop. Read it silently several times. Then apply the strategy that was developed in the previous exercises in this lesson.

Strategy for Telling a Story

- ■ Locate the problem words

- ■ Diagram the problem words

- ■ Practice the problem words

- ■ Mark all pitch jumps

- ■ Mark all ligatures

- ■ Mark all blends

- ■ Practice

- ■ Tell the story

Andy was lost. No mouse should get lost. Andy was an intelligent mouse who knew his way around the woods. But he was lost. When he entered a cave to rest, he didn't see the lion who was asleep in the corner. He didn't even see the name of the lion above the entrance—Ivan the Awful. His name said it all. Ivan was awful. In fact, Andy didn't realize that he was sitting on the lion's tail. He thought it was a comfortable rock.

All of a sudden the mighty Ivan awoke. Andy tried to run for cover. Before he could move, the great lion's paw came down on him. Ivan the Awful was about to end

Andy's life. The smart little mouse cried, "Mr. Lion, please don't eat me. I lost my way and didn't know I entered your house. I am too small to satisfy your hunger." Ivan the Awful looked at Andy and realized that the mouse was right. He was too small to eat. In a friendly mood, the king of all the animals let the tiny mouse go.

Some time later, while hunting in the woods, Ivan fell into a trap. The heavy ropes held him, just as he himself had held the tiny Andy. The lion gave a loud roar that was heard by all the animals in the forest. Andy, who was playing in the woods, heard the roar. He recognized it as that of his good friend Ivan. He eagerly ran to the place where the mighty animal was held by the ropes. Andy's teeth were very sharp, so he quickly chewed through the knot. Soon Ivan the Awful was free. He learned that a little mouse could return a big favor.

The moral of the story is: An act of kindness is a good investment.

EXERCISE 11. A Personal Story

Write a very short story about an experience you have had. Prepare it for presentation. You might select a vacation trip, a famous story that you can tell in your own words, a humorous story, or some imaginary story that you have made up. Use the strategy that you have learned.

_____

_____

_____

_____

_____

_____

_____

_____

_____

_____

_____

_____

_____

_____

_____

_____

_____

_____

LESSON 17

Speaking in Formal Situations

OBJECTIVE

In this lesson, we will learn how to prepare formal presentations for those times when you will be called upon to speak in public. There is a difference between informal conversational speech, telling a story to a group, and a formal public presentation. Speaking to the Board of Directors of a company, giving a speech at a business luncheon, teaching a class, and delivering a research paper at a convention are examples of public speaking. We wil also practice *extemporaneous talking* for use in situations that permit little or no time for preparation.

INSTRUCTOR'S NOTES FOR LESSON 17

Materials and Preclass Preparation

1. Transparency of the strategy for preparing a formal speech.
2. Tourist information regarding the community (from telephone books, Chamber of Commerce, the American Automobile Association, and so on).
3. A telephone.
4. Announcements or advertisements from the newspaper.

Concepts

1. Compare the strategy for formal presentations to that used for telling a story (Lesson 16). Discuss what the differences and similarities are with students.
2. Although formal presentations do not have to be long, they do need to be controlled.
3. For the formal 5–7 minute presentation, students should be advised to select a topic that is relevant to their work, study, or life situation, not something that will require extended study and research.
4. Students should be reminded of the purpose of this lesson—to develop control in formal situations. They will frequently let the topic dominate their behavior and forget why they are doing these things. This is not a speech class, but a class in presentation form.

Exercises

1. (Exercise 1a, 1b, and 1c) In the first part of this activity, students will gather information about a place of interest. Then they will use the information to (a) answer questions and (b) make a short presentation about their topic. Remind students that they are using a strategy to do what they are doing.
2. (Exercise 2) After the students have prepared their announcements, it might be interesting to role play by using video equipment to record or a tape recorder. Continue to monitor sentence structure and grammar.
3. (Exercise 3) This self-explanatory exercise is the central focus for this lesson. It is what the previous exercises have been developing. Make sure that students are taken through each step.
4. (Exercise 4) The questions are presented in the student's book to control some of the initial anxiety. In other words, if they so desire, students may prepare for this exercise by thinking about each of the five questions. Remind students that control is important.
5. (Exercise 5) Here are some questions that you may use (or ideas for questions that you may ask):

    What are the three best (worst) things about your job/major?

    Why should a person visit this city/state on a vacation?

    Are taxes fair?

    What are the advantages/disadvantages of . . .

    a liberal education?

    a brand new car?

    your own home?

    winning the lottery?

    using credit cards?

    How important is it to travel to many places?

    Who is the most important person in world history?

    Should there be . . .

    a universal language?

    a universal monetary system?

    one world government?

    Other topics: current political leaders, current problems on campus or in the community, disasters, the environment, health care, aging.

A STRATEGY FOR PREPARING A FORMAL SPEECH

Many things about speaking in public are the same as when we are speaking conversationally. We continue to (1) practice technical or difficult words, (2) use standard intonation, and (3) mark all ligatures and blends as appropriate for the sentences that we are saying. We also communicate our ideas with interest and emotion, as we do when speaking to a good friend. In fact, everything that you have learned in this text is applicable to speaking formally in public.

Yet, there is a major difference. If you are speaking formally, you must speak with sufficient loudness to be heard by the person in the last seat in the room. In conversational speech, it is important to speak with just enough loudness to be heard. In public speaking, the loudness level that we use is much greater. However, the use of pitch is *not* replaced by loudness. Not only must we speak to be heard, we must continue to *walk, jump, step*, and *fall*. Combining these two speech elements (Lesson 2) requires practice. Therefore, we need a strategy to use in preparing to speak in public.

Strategy: Here is the most efficient way to prepare for a speech.

1. Write the speech or decide what you are going to say.
2. Practice the new or difficult words.
3. Decide where you are going to jump in pitch.
4. Mark all of the ligatures.
5. Mark all of the blends.
6. Practice by using your marked script.
7. Deliver the speech with sufficient loudness to be heard by everyone.

EXERCISE 1. Discovering Your Community

a. Finding Information

Your local Chamber of Commerce or telephone book has a wealth of information on places to visit in your city, state, or elsewhere. Your teacher will help you to select a place you have visited or would like to visit. Write at least two responses for each of these questions. Keep your sentences short for greater control. Decide what the important words are so that you can *walk, jump, step*, and *fall* appropriately.

■ Why did (or could) you select this particular place to visit?

■ Where is it located? What is its address?

■ What is its telephone number?

■ When is the place open (days of the week and hours)?

■ What will you see when you go there? (List several things, if possible.)

■ Why should everyone visit this place?

b. Role-playing: Talking on the Telephone

Another person will ask for information based on the questions in Exercise 1a, and will "call you on the telephone." Respond appropriately.

c. Formal Presentation

Write a formal speech in which you try to convince your listener(s) to visit the place that you have selected. Include the information from Exercise 1a.

EXERCISE 2. An Important Announcement

Obtain a newspaper and locate an article or advertisement about a concert, meeting, film, play, or other event that will soon be presented in your community. Prepare a short announcement in which you answer these questions: Who? What? Where? When? Why? How much? Present your announcement.

EXERCISE 3. Preparing a Formal Speech

Frequently, we have to make a public presentation on some topic of interest to us. This activity will provide you with an opportunity to educate your listener(s) on something that you understand and have prepared. Your speech should be 5–7 minutes in length.

Step 1: Decide on what you want to do. Here are some options:

   a. If you are a teacher, present part of a lecture.

   b. If you work with small groups, describe a picture, or a series of pictures that tell a story.

   c. If you work for a company, tell about the work that you do.

   d. Provide technical information based on your expertise.

e. Introduce a hobby, sport, or artwork.

f. Talk about your major or a school that you attend(ed).

g. Persuade your listener(s) to do something.

    (1) Describe a problem.

    (2) Present a solution to a problem.

    (3) Persuade your listener(s) to see a problem differently.

Step 2: Plan the content of what you are going to say. You might have to read, take notes, think, or outline.

a. Start with general information and then gradually add specifics.

b. Start with facts and then gradually add opinion.

c. Start with what is known and then gradually add what is doubtful.

d. Use vocabulary that is understood and then gradually add special vocabulary.

e. Use visuals or demonstrations, if appropriate.

Step 3: Work on delivery. Review the *strategy* at the beginning of this lesson.

a. Write or outline your speech, especially the introduction and the conclusion.

b. Decide what words you are going to use. Practice the pronunciation of technical or difficult words.

c. Where are you going to jump? More than once? How will you step down and fall?

d. Mark and practice all ligatures and blends.

e. Practice your speech again and again.

Step 4: Present your speech.

a. Look at your audience as you speak.

b. Speak loudly enough to be heard by the person in the last row.

EXTEMPORANEOUS TALKING

A prepared formal presentation provides time for thinking about what we are going to say and how we are going to say it. We also have time to practice the speech until it is understandable. However, most of the speaking that we do, both formal and informal, is *extemporaneous*, spontaneous talking done without much time for preparation. We think about what we are going to say, not *how* we are going to say it. For this reason, the principles taught in this text must be learned *very* well because there is not much time to think about *how* you are going to speak when you speak extemporaneously. If you have not practiced the lessons in this text sufficiently, your *interlanguage accent* (see Lesson 2) will probably be most difficult to understand whenever you speak extemporaneously. Therefore, extemporaneous talking provides the best test of success in accent modification.

EXERCISE 4. Questions to Answer

To prepare for extemporaneous talking (Exercise 5), your teacher will ask you one or more of these questions. You will have 3 minutes to *think about* what you want to say. Then you will have 1 or 2 minutes to present your main ideas. If possible, make a tape recording of your answer so that you can analyze your use of standard intonation and special emphasis.

Question 1. As a result of this class, what have you learned about the pronunciation of American English?

Question 2. What advice would you give to a person from your country who wants to come to the United States to study American English?

Question 3. Why, in your opinion, is it so difficult to speak another language?

Question 4. How is an extemporaneous speech different from a formal speech?

Question 5. What are the most important steps in the strategy for preparing a formal speech?

EXERCISE 5. Answering Questions Extemporaneously

Your teacher will ask you some more questions which you will answer without any time for preparation. If possible, make a tape recording of your answer so that you can analyze your use of standard intonation and special emphasis.

LESSON 18

Offering Choices

OBJECTIVE

This lesson will help you use appropriate intonation for questions that offer the listener a choice. The intonation pattern used for offering choices combines the upward steps of yes/no questions and the step down, fall of information-asking questions and most sentences.

QUESTIONS THAT OFFER A CHOICE

Sometimes we want to offer our listener a choice between two things, an option to select one thing or the other. One way to do this is to ask two yes/no questions as in this example.

Example: Two Yes/No Questions

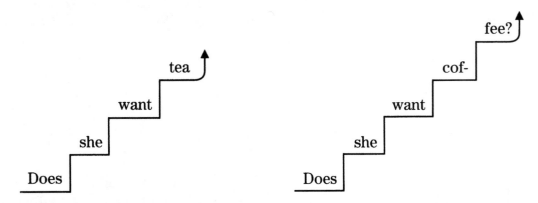

These questions are both asked with a step up in pitch on each syllable to the end of the question, that is, on *tea* and on the final syllable of *coffee*. However, when these two yes/no questions are combined to offer a choice to the listener, the intonation for the *first* choice follows the same pattern of upward steps in pitch that applies to yes/no questions in general. The intonation for the *second* choice steps down to the end and falls on the last syllable, in the manner used for information-asking questions and standard intonation. See *Figure 18–1*. The first choice is usually connected to the second choice by the word *or* as in this example.

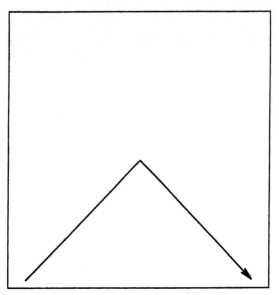

Figure 18–1. Choice question intonation. Intonation for these questions results from combining yes/no question and information-asking question intonation.

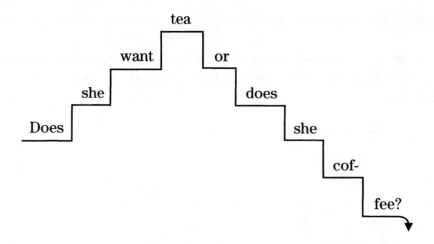

EXERCISE 1. Making Choice Questions

Say these pairs of sentences with usual yes/no (upward) question intonation. Then combine the sentences with *or* and step down and fall in pitch on the second choice.

Example: Does she want tea?
Does she want coffee?
Does she want tea or does she want coffee?

1. **(a)** Will we study? **(b)** Will we go to the movies?

2. **(a)** Should she do her homework? **(b)** Should she visit her mother?

3. **(a)** Is it going to rain? **(b)** Is it going to snow?

4. **(a)** Do you want to step up in pitch? **(b)** Do you want to step down?

5. **(a)** Are they on vacation? **(b)** Are they sick?

6. **(a)** Is she single? **(b)** Is she married?

7. **(a)** Can you work on Saturday? **(b)** Can you work on Monday?

8. **(a)** Are you going to California? **(b)** Are you going to Florida?

EXERCISE 2. How to Shorten Choice Questions

You can shorten these questions by omitting the repeated words. For example, *Will we study or will we go to the movies?* can become, *Will we study or go to the movies?* by omitting the second set of repeated (underlined) words. The same procedures apply for stepping up on the first choice and stepping down and falling on the second choice, even when the question is shortened. Return to Exercise 1 and practice the choice questions with the *short* form.

Example: Does she want tea or coffee?

EXERCISE 3. Shortened Choice Questions

Practice these questions that offer a choice.

1. Do you want to play **voll**eyball or basketball?

2. Is dinner at **six** or seven o'clock?

3. Can they join us for **lunch** or dinner?

4. Will the class be offered **this** term or next?

5. Did the team **win** or lose?

EXERCISE 4. Asking Questions that Offer Two Choices

Here is list of choices. Ask a choice question that can be answered by either of the words in Columns **A** and **B** (we will use Column **C** later). Remember that we can make regular yes/no questions from each choice: *Is the appointment for Thursday? (Yes/No); Is the appointment for Friday? (Yes/No).* We can also ask a longer choice question: *Is the appointment for Thursday or is the appointment for Friday?* However, the short version—*Is the appointment for Thursday or Friday?*—is always preferred.

Example: **A**   **B**   **C**

Thursday   Friday   Saturday

Is the appointment for Thursday or Friday?

Diagram:

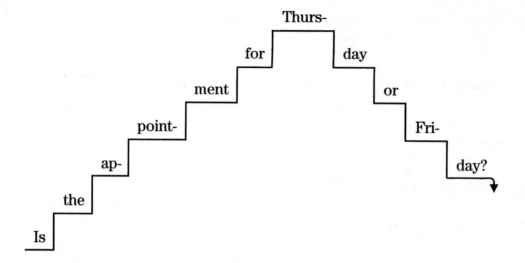

> *Pronunciation Note:* Many speakers of American English will make choice questions by walking on average pitch (with no steps) on *Is the appointment for*, followed by the pitch jump on the first syllable of *Thursday*, with steps down on each syllable thereafter and a fall on the last syllable. You may use either form in these exercises.

	A	B	C
1.	coffee	tea	milk
2.	Gary's	Roger's	Tom's
3.	Alice	Mary	Jane
4.	Master's	Doctor's	Bachelor's (degree)
5.	June	July	August
6.	turkey	chicken	ham
7.	Spain	Italy	Portugal
8.	newspaper	radio	television
9.	McDonald's	Wendy's	Burger King

10. small	medium	large
11. twenty dollars	thirty dollars	forty dollars
12. an actor	a musician	a dancer

INFORMATION-ASKING QUESTIONS WITH TWO CHOICES

EXERCISE 5. Offering Choices with Information-Asking Questions

We can also offer choices by using information-asking questions. Remember to jump two times in these questions as shown by the words or syllables in **boldface** type.

1. **Who's** getting married, **Barb** or Ken?

2. **Where** are they going, to **Chi**na or Japan?

3. **How** much did you pay, **for**ty or fifty dollars?

4. **When** is the meeting, **Thurs**day or Friday?

5. **Which** way do you turn, **left** or right?

EXERCISE 6. Practice in Offering Choices

In this exercise, make up a question starting with a Wh- word. Follow usual step down intonation on the question after jumping on the Wh- word. Then, using the words in Columns **B** and **C** from Exercise 4, offer choices by jumping in pitch on the first choice and stepping down on the second choice. Fall on the last syllable.

Example (based on the example in Exercise 4):

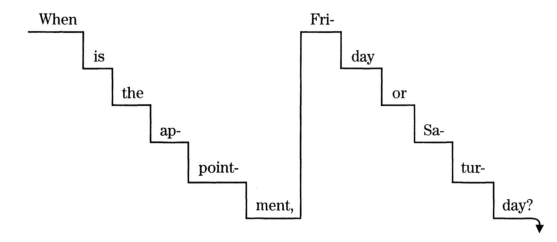

Continue offering choices with other Wh- words, such as *Who, Where, When, How much, Which, Whose,* and *What*.

QUESTIONS THAT PROVIDE SEVERAL CHOICES

We may want to provide our listener with more than two choices. For these times, we can use *list intonation* as discussed in Lesson 15. Study this example.

Example:

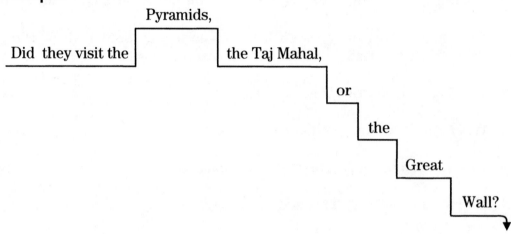

EXERCISE 7. Using List Intonation in Yes/No Questions

Practice these questions.

1. Do you like **watermelon**, cantaloupe, or bananas?

2. Is it a **Monday**, Wednesday, or Friday class?

3. Are they going to play **ping-pong**, chess, or checkers?

4. Will they leave **today**, tomorrow, or some other day?

5. Should we clean the **bedroom**, the family room, or the basement?

EXERCISE 8. Using List Intonation in Choice Questions

Practice asking questions that provide several choices by using the words in Columns **A, B,** and **C** from Exercise 4.

Example:

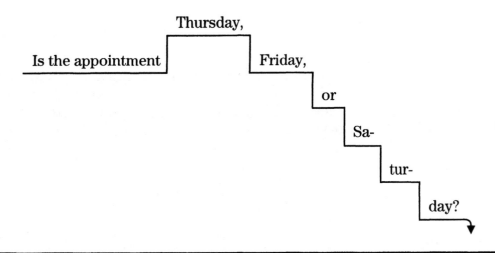

Thursday,

Is the appointment

Friday,

or

Sa-

tur-

day?

Exercise 9. Making Choice Questions

a. In this exercise, select a question word (the *do* verb) from those provided "1". Then select an appropriate subject (pronoun) word "2". Use the choices provided "3" to complete the question. First, ask questions that offer only two choices (**A** and **B**). Then use Column **C** to practice *list intonation* in multiple choice questions.

Example: 1. Question Word (Select One): Do/Does

        2. Subject Word (Select One): I/she/they

        3. Choices:

Verb	A	B	C
play	piano	organ	harp

Two-Choice Question: Do they play piano or organ?

Three-Choice Question (with *list intonation*): Do they play piano, organ, or harp?

1. Question Word (Select One): Do/Does/Did

2. Subject Word (Select One): he/she/they/you

3. Choices:

Verb	A	B	C
need	a coat	a sweater	a jacket
want	a car	a boat	a van
cook	beef	pork	turkey
paint	the house	the shed	the fence
prepare	a meal	a snack	a salad
write	a poem	a letter	an essay
discover	a lake	an island	a river

visit	the zoo	the museum	the park
refinish	the chair	the table	the desk
turn off	the radio	the VCR	the television

b. Continue as above by selecting a question word (the *be* verb) from those provided in "1," then choosing a subject (or pronoun) word from "2." Finally, use the choices provided in "3" to complete the question. First, ask questions that offer only two choices (**A** and **B**). Then use Column **C** to practice *list intonation* in multiple choice questions.

1. Question Word (Select One): Is/Was/Are/Were

2. Subject Word (Select One): he/she/it/they/you

3. Choices:

A	B	C
from New York	from Philadelphia	from San Francisco
sick	well	worse than yesterday
blue	green	red
happy	sad	just OK
hungry	thirsty	famished
going to the movie	the play	the concert
married	single	divorced
a freshman	a sophomore	a junior
a student	a teacher	an administrator
from China	from Korea	from Russia

c. Continue as above by selecting a question word (the *have* verb) from those provided in "1," then choosing a subject (or pronoun) word from "2." Finally, use the choices provided in "3" to complete the question. First, ask questions that offer only two choices (**A** and **B**). Then use Column **C** to practice *list intonation* in multiple choice questions.

1. Question Word (Select One): Have/Has

2. Subject Word (Select One): you/they/she/he

3. Choices:

Verb	A	B	C
eaten	cake	ice cream	pie
gone to	the zoo	the museum	the park
seen	the play	the movie	the concert
—	read the book	seen the play	gone to the movie
finished	the homework	the review	the termpaper
written	to Mary	to John	to Alice
cleaned	the stove	the sink	the refrigerator
made	the cakes	the pies	the punch
painted	the tables	the chairs	the desks
—	telephoned Mary	written to her	seen her recently

visited	Chicago	Kansas City	Tulsa
built	a fence	a deck	a doghouse

d. Continue as above by selecting a question word (the *do* verb) from those provided in "1," then choosing a subject (or pronoun) word from "2." Finally, use the choices provided in "3" to complete the question. First, ask questions that offer only two choices (**A** and **B**). Then use Column **C** to practice *list intonation* in multiple choice questions.

1. **Question Word** (Select One): Do/Does/Did

2. **Subject Word** (Select One): he/she/they/you

3. **Choices:**

A	**B**	**C**
mow the lawn	trim the hedge	water the garden
go to the bank	mail the letters	visit your mother
play tennis	swim laps	shoot baskets
go to the library	walk in the park	shop in the mall
drive your car	take a bus	travel by train
work in an office	teach school	sell insurance

EXERCISE 10. Writing Various Kinds of Choice Questions

a. Write three <u>two-choice</u> questions (*Is the appointment Thursday or Friday?*)

_____

_____

_____

b. Write three <u>information-asking two-choice</u> questions (*When is the appointment, Thursday or Friday?*).

_____

_____

_____

c. Write three choice questions with list intonation (*Is the appointment Thursday, Friday, or Saturday?*).

_____

_____

_____

OPEN-ENDED TWO-CHOICE QUESTIONS

Open-ended choice questions provide an opportunity for our listener to make a personal choice, one that is different from those we have offered. Some two-choice questions may be open-ended. Suppose that we think the appointment is for Thursday, but we could be wrong. We could ask, *Is the appointment for Thursday or some other day?* Using a variation of this open-ended choice, we could ask, *Do you want coffee or something else?* On other occasions, the last choice may suggest the opposite of the first choice. A negative phrase such as . . . *or not?* may be used. For example, we can ask, *Are you finished or not?* The intonation remains the same for these as for all two-choice questions.

OPEN-ENDED QUESTIONS THAT PROVIDE SEVERAL CHOICES

In asking open-ended questions that provide several choices, a vague phrase such as . . . *or something else?* may be used as the last choice. For example, we could ask, *Do you want coffee, tea, or something else?* using list intonation. As always, we step down on each syllable of the open-ended choice and fall on the last syllable.

EXERCISE 11. Playing the Who Am I? Game with Various Kinds of Choice Questions

Replay the question game from Lesson 11, Exercise 5, but use choice questions only, including open-ended choice questions.

Example: The name selected is *Mahatma Gandhi* (not known by the other players)

Question 1: *Are you a female or a male?* Answer: *Male.*

Question 2: *Are you alive or dead?* Answer: *Dead.*

Question 3: *Were you a leader or not?* Answer: *A leader.*

The game continues until . . .

Last Question: *Are you Mahatma Gandhi or someone else?*
Answer: *I'm Mahatma Gandhi.*

The student guessing correctly becomes "it" for the next round.

LESSON 19

Asking Questions With Tags

OBJECTIVE

This lesson, you will learn how to ask a different kind of yes/no question. It is known as a *tag question* because the part that asks the question is "tagged on" to the end of a sentence. Intonation on the tag varies with the intent of the speaker

---

ASKING TAG QUESTIONS

You know what tag questions are, don't you? This question is an example of a tag question. The question begins with a statement (*You know what tag questions are*) with the question "tagging along behind" or attached at the end (*don't you?*). Here are some other examples:

You are going to the party, aren't you?

Tom's not your brother, is he?

Mary wrote to her family, didn't she?

You don't need to borrow my car, do you?

Remember that tag questions are made by making a statement (a sentence) and then adding a question at the end:

SENTENCE + TAG

If the sentence is **AFFIRMATIVE**, make the tag **NEGATIVE**.

Mister Fox was just about famished, wasn't he?

If the sentence is **NEGATIVE**, make the tag **AFFIRMATIVE**.

Mister Fox couldn't reach the grapes, could he?

INTONATION FOR TAG QUESTIONS

On the surface, tag questions appear to be an easy way to ask questions. However, we have to learn to vary our use of standard *walk, jump, step, fall* intonation, depending on our intent. Here are the principles (Avery & Ehrlich, 1992). See *Figure 19–1.*

1. Use standard (or special emphasis) intonation on the sentence part of the question. *Mister Fox was **just** about famished . . .*

2. If you *do not know the answer* and want the listener to answer *yes* or *no, step up* in pitch on the tag as for yes/no questions.

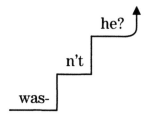

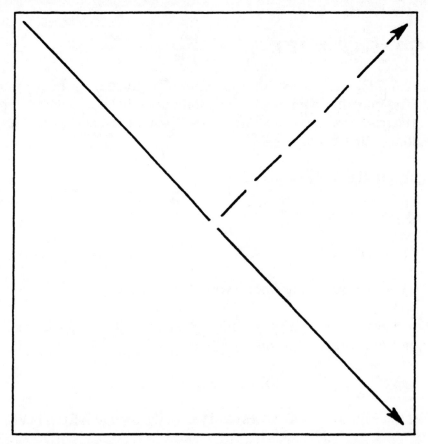

Figure 19–1. Tag question intonation. This figure shows the pitch jump, step down, and fall (standard intonation) used for the sentence portion of the tag question. The tag is produced by a rising (yes/no) intonation or a falling (information-asking) intonation.

3. If you *think you know the answer* and expect *agreement or confirmation* from the listener, *step down* in pitch on the tag and fall on the last syllable.

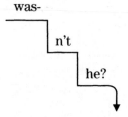

Therefore, in the question, *Tom's not your brother, is he?* if you *do not know the answer* and are asking your listener to respond with *yes* or *no*, you step up on the tag.

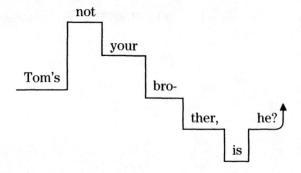

In the question, *You're going to the party, aren't you?* if you *expect your listener to agree with you*, step down and fall on the tag.

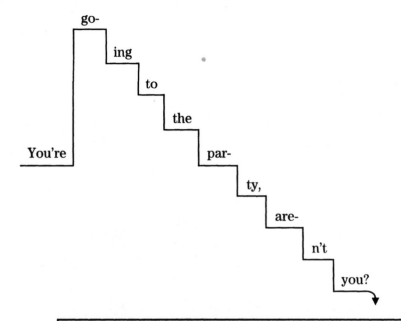

> *Pronunciation Note:* Speakers of American English may jump in pitch on the first syllable of the tag (*aren't*) if the sentence before the tag is long. In any event, the tag still steps and falls if the speaker expects agreement from the listener.

EXERCISE 1. Asking Tag Questions When You Do Not Know the Answer

Make the following statements into tag questions that require a *yes* or *no* from your listener. Use standard intonation on the sentence portion of the question and step up in pitch on the tag.

1. You know the answer.

2. Your sister is here.

3. Jane should call me later.

4. I can't help it.

5. He won't be late.

6. The reservations are ready.

7. We don't want a car.

8. He accepted the job.

9. Today is Monday.

10. Jim went home.

11. Sue doesn't want a ride.

12. Mary and Sam are getting married.

13. The electricity went off.

14. My mother didn't call.

15. The trip has been canceled.

16. They didn't win the game.

17. You know how to make a telephone call.

18. They always watch TV on Friday nights.

19. I can't remember everything.

20. Bill doesn't work in the library on weekends.

EXERCISE 2. Making Tag Questions When You Expect Agreement

Using the same sentences as in Exercise 1, make tag questions in which you expect your listener to agree with your initial statement or sentence. Step down and fall on the tag.

EXERCISE 3. Testing Your Ability to Make Proper Tags

For this exercise, before you ask a tag question, decide whether you want agreement or information from your listener, and practice asking tag questions. Use the sentences in Exercise 1. Did your listener answer appropriately?

EXERCISE 4. Playing the *Who Am I?* Game with Tag Questions

Replay the question games from Lesson 11, Exercise 5 and Lesson 18, Exercise 11, but use tag questions only.

Example: The name selected is Mahatma Gandhi (not known by the other players)

Question 1: *You're a female, aren't you?*   Answer: *No.*

(Step up on the tag because you don't know the answer.)

Question 2: *You are alive, aren't you?*   Answer: *No.*

Question 3: *You were a leader, weren't you?*   Answer: *Yes.*

The game continues until . . .

Last Question: *You're Mahatma Gandhi, aren't you?*   Answer: *Yes.*

(Step down and fall on the tag because you think you know the answer and expect agreement.)

The student guessing correctly becomes "it" for the next round.

LESSON 20

Review of Standard Intonation and Its Variations

OBJECTIVE

In this lesson, we will review the common sentence types that have been introduced and studied in this text. Throughout this course of study, there have not been many sentence patterns to memorize. You have seen that once standard sentence intonation is established, all other patterns are variations on this *walk, jump, step, fall* sequence.

STANDARD INTONATION

In American English, the standard intonation pattern is *walk* in average pitch to an important word, usually early in the sentence and *jump* in pitch on the prominent (stressed) syllable of that word. Then *step* down in pitch to the end of the sentence, ending with a *fall* in pitch on the last syllable. See Lessons 2 to 6 and 8.

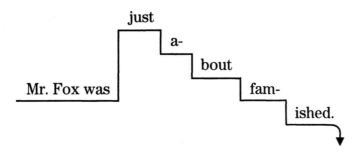

Examples: They **are**n't going to the picnic.

John **al**ways does his work.

She gave a **won**derful report.

SPECIAL EMPHASIS INTONATION

It is possible to jump in pitch on any important word or words in a sentence because of their special meaning. This is called *special emphasis*. Use it carefully. The words you jump up on should be very important to your message. In this example, the jump in pitch may occur on the word written in **boldface** type. Notice how the emphasis of the sentence changes when the pitch jump is changed. See Lesson 12.

Examples: **Give** Pam some cake.

Give **Pam** some cake.

Give Pam **some** cake.

Give Pam some **cake**.

INTONATION FOR INFORMATION-ASKING QUESTIONS

Jump in pitch on the Wh- word and step down on each syllable that follows, with a fall in pitch on the last syllable. This pattern is also used for sentences that are not information-asking questions (**Jim** lives in the dorm.). See Lesson 7.

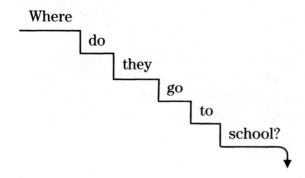

Examples: **Which** computer should I buy?

When is your birthday?

Where do you work?

YES/NO QUESTION INTONATION

Standard intonation is reversed for questions that may be answered with a *yes* or *no*. Start below average pitch and step up on every syllable that follows to the end of the question. See Lesson 11.

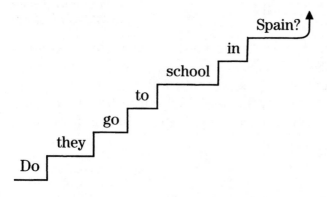

Examples: Are they waiting for **us**?

Am I saying it **right**?

Can you travel during the holi**days**?

INTONATION IN LONGER SENTENCES

A thought expressed in one sentence may be combined with another thought to produce a longer sentence. When thoughts are combined, it may be necessary to jump in pitch more than one time. See Lesson 15.

■ **Contrasting Information.** When words contrast in a longer sentence, the pitch jump may occur on each contrasting word. In this example, the pitch jump may be used to contrast the two people (*Jim* and *Julie*) or even the two activities (*washed* and *dried*).

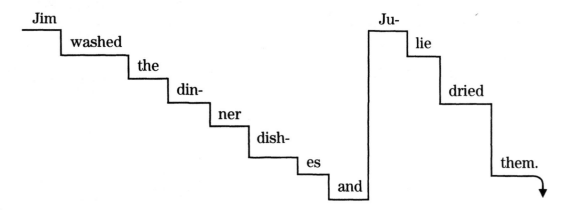

Examples: **Mr.** Smith wanted to stay home but his **child**ren wanted to take a vacation.

This biology class works hard, but **that** one works harder.

I for**got** to bring enough money, so I had to **bor**row some.

■ **Statements.** When two sentences are joined together with connecting words such as *and, but, or, so, when,* or *although,* then *both* sentences may have a pitch jump.

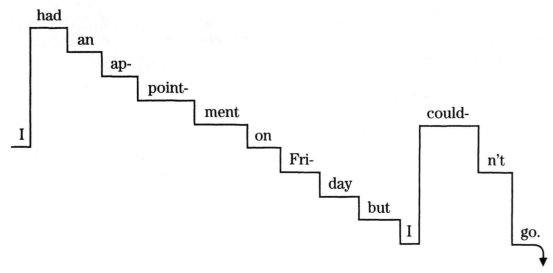

Examples: I'd **like** to learn several other languages, but I'm **too** busy.

We were **loo**king through an old book, and a **twen**ty-dollar bill fell to the floor.

Jane went to the store so she could **buy** some more apples.

■ **List Intonation.** For a list of items, standard intonation is used with one minor change — each item in the list is said on a different pitch level but without any intermediate steps on the syllables. In this example, the pitch jump occurs on the first syllable of *Pyramids*, but with no step down in pitch until the first syllable of *the Taj Mahal*, again with no step down until the entire item is said. Then we step down on *the Great*, and fall on *Wall*. In short, stay on the same pitch level through each item on the list until the last item. Then step down and fall as usual.

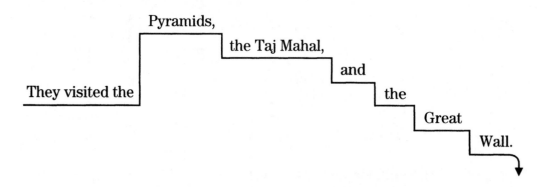

Examples: They wanted a **house**, a car, and a boat.

Our school has **baseball**, football, soccer, and bowling teams.

We plan to visit **Delaware**, Maryland, and Virginia.

CHOICE QUESTION INTONATION

When a question offers a choice between two things, step up on the first choice as for as yes/no question, and step down on the second choice to the final fall on the last syllable. See Lesson 18.

■ **Two Choices—Yes/No Questions**

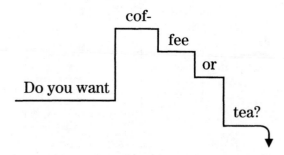

Examples: Do you want to play **vol**leyball or basketball?

Is dinner at **six** or seven o'clock?

Can they join us for **lunch** or dinner?

■ Two Choices—Information-asking Questions

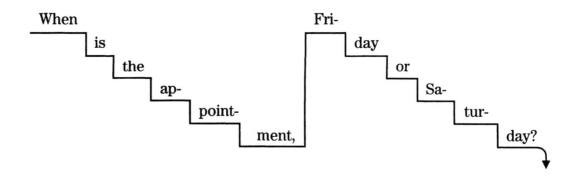

Examples: **Who's** getting married, **Barb** or Ken?

Where are they going, to **Chi**na or Japan?

How much did you pay, **for**ty or fifty dollars?

■ More Than Two Choices—Yes/No Questions (List Intonation)

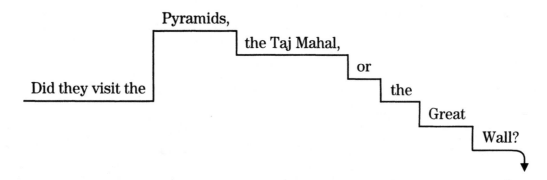

Examples: Do you like **watermelon**, cantaloupe, or bananas?

Is it a **Monday**, Wednesday, or Friday class?

Are they going to play **ping-pong**, chess, or checkers?

TAG QUESTION INTONATION

If the sentence is affirmative, make the tag negative. If the sentence is negative, make the tag affirmative. Use *walk, jump, step, fall* intonation on the sentence and (a) if you want an answer to the tag, step up; and (b) if you want your listener to agree with you, step down and fall on the tag. See Lesson 19.

■ You Want an Answer

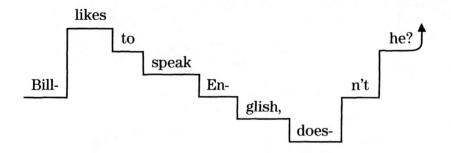

Examples: Your **sis**ter is here, isn't **she**?

He ac**cep**ted the job, didn't **he**?

Sue **does**n't need a ride, does **she**?

■ **You Expect Agreement**

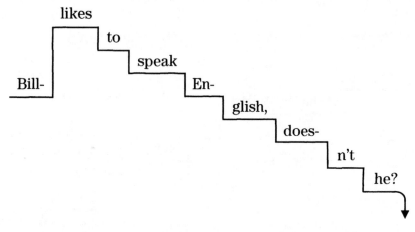

Examples: Your **sis**ter is here, isn't she?

He ac**cep**ted the job, didn't he?

Sue **does**n't need a ride, does she?

REVIEW OF THE VARIATIONS OF STANDARD INTONATION FOR QUESTIONS

Figure 20–1 represents a review of question intonation.

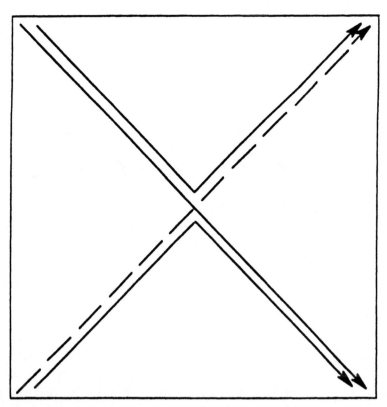

Figure 20–1. Question intonation review. The downward line represents information-asking questions (Lesson 7) and tag questions (Lesson 19) in which we expect agreement. The dashed upward line represents yes/no question intonation (Lesson 11). The "V" line at the top is used in tag question intonation (Lesson 19) when we need information. The inverted "V" at the bottom is used in choice question intonation (Lesson 18).

REVIEW ACTIVITIES

ACTIVITY 1. Revising Your Philosophy Statement

Review the philosophy of accent modification that you wrote in Lesson 1. How would you write your philosophy statement now? What would you change? What would you leave the same?

_____

_____

_____

_____

_____

_____

_____

_____

Activity 2. Reviewing Your *Pronunciation Notebook*

Turn to your *Pronunciation Notebook*. How many of the words and phrases that you included have become part of your everyday vocabulary? Are you still pronouncing them as you diagrammed them in your *Notebook*? Continue to add words and phrases as you progress in accent modification.

Activity 3. Setting Goals for Continued Growth in Accent Modification

Review your personal goals and objectives from your *Accent Modification Agreement*. List your areas of improvement. Then list those things that you must continue to work on—your goals for improvement. You know by now that accent modification requires constant attention. How do you plan to obtain your goals for continued progress?

a. Areas of Progress: _____

_____

_____

_____

b. Goals: _____

_____

_____

_____

c. Plan: _____

_____

_____

TEN THINGS TO REMEMBER

1. Don't go back to the "old you"—to your old way of speaking. You will be tempted because it is the "easy" thing to do. Don't forget, if the way you usually speak sounds understandable to you, it may not be understandable to others; if it sounds natural to you, it may sound unnatural to others.

2. Modifying your accent requires constant attention, but you now have the tools to be successful.

3. Pitch is the most important speech element in American English. Use it whenever you speak.

4. Remember to use standard intonation —

Walk, Jump, Step, Fall

5. Use continuous airflow on /th/ and /TH/ and interrupted airflow on /p/ and /b/.

6. Round your lips slightly to produce the American English /r/, /sh/, /zh/, /ch/, and /j/ sounds. The lips are rounded tightly for the /w/ sound. No lip rounding is used for /l/ and /v/.

7. Continue to work on ligatures and blends until they occur naturally.

8. The "golden rule" of accent modification is to speak to your listener the way you want your listener to speak to you.

9. Periodically, go over the exercises in this text and the accompanying audio cassettes.

10. Look for opportunities to practice what you have learned every day.

References

Avery, P., & Ehrlich, S. (1992). *Teaching American English pronunciation.* Oxford: Oxford University Press.

Bolinger, D. (1986). *Intonation and parts: Melody in spoken English.* Stanford, CA: Stanford University Press.

Edwards, H. (1992). *Applied phonetics: The sounds of American English.* San Diego, CA: Singular Publishing Group.

Goldman-Eisler, F. (1968). *Psycholinguistics: Experiments in spontaneous speech.* New York: Academic Press.

Heilman, A. (1993). *Phonics in proper perspective* (7th ed.). New York: Macmillan.

Random House Webster's dictionary. (1991). New York: Random House.

Selinker, L. (1972). Interlanguage. *International Review of Applied Linguistics, 10,* 209–231.

Stern, D. (1991). *Breaking the accent barrier* (video). Los Angeles: Video Language Products.

Temperley, M. (1987). Linking and deletion in final consonant clusters. In J. Morley (Ed.), *Current perspectives on pronunciation* (pp. 59–82). Washington, DC: Teachers of English to Speakers of Other Languages, Inc.

APPENDIX A

Student Questionnaire

Name_____Age_____Sex_____

Major (if in school)_____ Home Phone_____

Future/Present Career_____

Current Employment _____ Work Phone_____

TOEFL or other ESL Test Score_____ Name of Test if different from TOEFL

_____

What country do you come from? _____

What is your first (or native) language? _____

   Dialect, if different _____

What other languages do you speak? _____

If you speak another variety of English, which? _____

Did you study American English before coming to this country? Yes ☐   No ☐

How were you were taught English (check all that apply):

_____ reading/writing/listening	_____ by native English teachers
_____ grammar/vocabulary/translation	_____ by nonnative English teachers
_____ self-study	_____ in elementary school
_____ by radio/TV	_____ in high school
_____ in English class	_____ in college
_____ ESL class	_____ by talking to English speakers
_____ intensive language school	_____ by family members
_____ other: _____	

For how many years have you **studied** English? _____

For how many years have you **spoken** English? _____

How many hours on an average day do you speak your native language? _____

How many hours on an average day do you speak English? _____

As a child, did you have any problems in learning or speaking your native language?

Yes ☐ No ☐   If Yes, please explain _____

_____

Do you have any hearing difficulties? Yes ☐ No ☐   If Yes, please explain:

_____

Speaking Opportunities. Here is a list of speaking situations. Tell how frequently you participate in each by using these numbers:

    1 — Never   2 — Rarely   3 — Sometimes   4 — Every day

Then tell the difficulty that each situation gives you by using these numbers:

0 — Not Applicable 1 — No difficulty 2 — Some difficulty 3 — Great difficulty

Situation	Frequency	Difficulty
Conversation with friends	_____	_____
Asking Questions	_____	_____
Responding to Questions	_____	_____
Presenting a Prepared Speech or Report	_____	_____
Tutoring or Small Group Discussion	_____	_____
Talking on the Telephone	_____	_____
Classroom Teaching	_____	_____
Presenting Plans/Proposals in Business Meetings	_____	_____

Listening Opportunities. Here is a list of listening situations. Tell how frequently you participate in each by using these numbers:

    1 — Never   **2 — Rarely**   **3 — Sometimes**   **4 — Every day**

Then tell the difficulty that each situation gives you by using these numbers:

0 — Not Applicable **1 — No difficulty** **2 — Some difficulty** **3 — Great difficulty**

Situation	Frequency	Difficulty
Radio, Television	____	____
Lectures	____	____
Business Meetings	____	____
Telephone Talk	____	____
Conversations	____	____
Understanding Questions	____	____

What other information will your teacher(s) need to know about you?

_____

_____

_____   _____

Signature   Date

APPENDIX B

Accent Modification Agreement

ACCENT MODIFICATION
AGREEMENT

FOR

_____

I. Introductory Statement

The success of Accent Modification is in your hands. The best techniques are useless unless they are put into practice daily.

II. General Goals of Accent Modification

1. To use the primary speech elements appropriately.

2. To use the secondary speech elements appropriately.

3. To use standard intonation appropriately.

4. To control the syllable appropriately in American English.

5. To produce understandable speech sounds.

6. To speak in a communicative manner.

III. Requirements for Obtaining the Goals

1. Attend every class.
2. Come to class prepared (homework complete and lessons studied).
3. Study the textbook, obtain a tape recorder, and practice with the audiocassettes.
4. Bring your textbook to every class.
5. Obtain a small pocket mirror and bring it to every class.
6. Practice your new knowledge when speaking with native speakers of American English.

IV. Individual Objectives (From Form 1b and Form 2b)

1. ___ I will raise___/lower___ my average pitch.
2. ___ I will increase___/decrease___ my pitch range.
3. ___ I will increase___/decrease___ my rate of speaking.
4. ___ I will increase___/decrease___ the level of my overall loudness.
5. ___ I will use appropriate pitch for emphasis in sentences instead of loudness___ or monotone speech___.

6. ___ I will use appropriate average pitch (walk) to the pitch jump.
7. ___ I will increase___/decrease___ the number of pitch jumps.
8. ___ I will use appropriate syllable/word for the pitch jump.
9. ___ I will use appropriate step down in pitch from the pitch jump in sentences by using steps___/smaller steps___.
10. ___ I will use appropriate fall in pitch at the ends of sentences; instead of an upward glide___
11. ___ I will increase___/decrease___ the number of pauses.
12. ___ I will pronounce the ends of words___; and not add extra syllables___ or sounds___.
13. ___ I will use ligatures and blends appropriately.
14. ___ I will speak in a more communicative manner.
15. ___ I will make my speech more understandable by modifying these processes:

___ avoid spelling pronunciations
___ greater use of the neutral vowel /ə/ (vowel reduction)
  •*Sound Process Errors (from Form 2b)*•
___ lip-rounding on /sh/, /zh/, /ch/, /j/, /r/, /w/
___ no lip-rounding on /l/ or /v/
___ continuous airflow on /th/, /TH/
___ improve placement of /th/ or /TH/
___ interrupted airflow on /p/, /b/
___ improve pronunciation of consonant clusters: With /r/___/ /l/___
___ increase vowel duration before voiced sounds,i.e., /z/, /d/, /g/

16. Other objectives: _____

I,_____, have read the above agreement and understand the necessity of setting goals for my accent modification during the _____course of study and beyond. I wish to comply with these goals and objectives and continue to work on the improvement of my speech.

Date _____

APPENDIX C

Pronunciation Notebook

WORD	DICTIONARY	DIAGRAM

WORD	DICTIONARY	DIAGRAM

WORD	DICTIONARY	DIAGRAM

WORD	DICTIONARY	DIAGRAM

APPENDIX D

The Pronunciation Alphabet Used in This Text

VOWELS			**CONSONANTS**		
ee	as in	bead	p	as in	pop
i	as in	bid	b	as in	Bob
a	as in	bay	t	as in	ten
e	as in	bed	d	as in	dad
ae	as in	bad	k, c	as in	kick
uw	as in	glue	g	as in	give
u	as in	good	f	as in	five
o	as in	go	v	as in	very
aw	as in	caught	th	as in	thin
ah	as in	cot	TH	as in	then
ə	as in	above	s	as in	see
yuw	as in	you	z	as in	zero
ai	as in	I	sh	as in	shop
ow	as in	now	zh	as in	vision
oi	as in	boy	h	as in	hat
ch	as in	chop	ng	as in	sing
j	as in	jar	r	as in	ring
m	as in	my	l	as in	let
n	as in	nine	w	as in	wet
			y	as in	yet

Index

R

Rate, 16, 18
Resonance, 14–15
Rhythm, 16
   duration, 159–163
   pausing, 159

S

Secondary speech elements, 17
Silent letters, pronunciation of, 177–179
Slight lip rounding, 29
Sound processes, 29
Special emphasis, 56, 151, 233
   longer sentences, 186
Speech elements, 15–17
Spelling
   guessing pronunciation from, 177–178
   principles, 177–179
Standard intonation, 51, 97, 151, 233, 239
   common mistakes, 52
   jump, step, fall, 33–34
   use of, 67–71
   walk, jump, fall, 36–37
   walk, jump, step, fall, 33–37
Step down, 54
Stepping down, critical second step, 84
Stress, 16
Structure words, 100
Syllable, 17–18, 171
   releasing sound, 18
   melodic sound, 18
Syllables
   deletion of, 179
   number of, 53

T

Tag questions, 225–227
   expecting confirmation, 226
   expecting information, 226–227
   intonation, in, 225–227, 237–239
   making, 225–227
   rules for, 225–227
Telling a story, 195
   strategy, 109, 199
Tongue placement, 45
Transfer, 9
Two–thought sentences, 183–184

V

Verbs, third person, 105, 107–108
Voiceless sounds, 13–14
Voicing, 13–14
Volume, 17
Vowels, 18–19

W

Walk, jump, step, fall, 51–52, 233, 239
   duration in, 159–161
   phrases and sentences, 67–71
Word endings
   past tense, 130–131, 147–148
   present/-s, 147–148
   -s, 105–108, 131

Y

Yes/no questions, 137, 211
   intonation, in, 234, 239